PSYCHIATRIC AND MENTAL HEALTH NURSING EDITION 6

ANNIE LAURIE CRAWFORD, M.Ed., R.N., F.A.A.N.

Formerly: Associate Professor, Psychiatric Nursing, Vanderbilt University School of Nursing; Director, Mental Health and Psychiatric Nursing Project, Southern Regional Education Board; Psychiatric Nursing Consultant, Florida State Board of Health; Institutions Nursing Supervisor, Department of Public Welfare, State of Minnesota; Director of Nurses, State Hospital South, Blackfoot, Idaho; Educational Director, Bangor State Hospital, Bangor Maine; Director of Nursing, Highland Hospital, Asheville, North Carolina

Recipient of the 1984 Distinguished Contribution to Psychiatric and Mental Health Nursing Award, presented by the Division on Psychiatric and Mental Health Nursing Practice of the American Nurses' Association

VIRGINIA CURRY KILANDER, M.Ed., R.N.

Formerly: Faculty, Mental Health, Gustavus Adolphus College Department of Nursing; Associate Professor, South Dakota State University, College of Nursing; Director, Mental Health and Psychiatric Nursing Pilot Project, Minnesota Department of Public Welfare; Instructor, Psychiatric Nursing, University of Minnesota School of Nursing

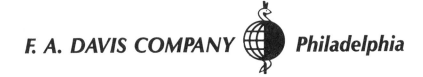

F. A. DAVIS COMPANY **Philadelphia**

Library of Congress Cataloging in Publication Data

Crawford, Annie Laurie.
  Psychiatric and mental health nursing.

  Rev. ed. of: Psychiatric nursing. 5th ed. 1980.
Includes bibliographies and index.
  1. Psychiatric nursing. I. Kilander, Virginia
Curry. II. Crawford, Annie Laurie. Psychiatric
nursing. III. Title. [DNLM: 1. Psychiatric
Nursing. WY 160 C899p]
RC440.C7 1985   610.73'68   84-11423
ISBN 0-8036-2113-2

PREFACE

The first edition (1954) of this publication was entitled *Nursing Manual for Psychiatric Aides*. It was designed to serve as a useful tool for instruction of the attendants, psychiatric aides, and technicians who were employed in the care of emotionally disturbed and mentally ill patients.

Succeeding editions, entitled *Psychiatric Nursing: A Basic Manual*, have been revised to reflect the changes in treatment programs, facilities, and services for patients. Vocational and technical schools preparing personnel for work with psychiatric patients have used and made suggestions for improvement in each succeeding edition.

The sixth edition is titled *Psychiatric and Mental Health Nursing*. It has been revised and expanded, and the format modified to reflect the need for a basic and more comprehensive text for vocational and technical nursing students and for the orientation and continuing education of staff members employed in the wide variety of agencies and institutions serving the needs of the special populations who use psychiatric and mental health services.

Four chapters prepared by contributors have been added. Their special interests, preparation, and current work uniquely qualify them to make these contributions. The authors believe these chapters substantially increase the value and usefulness of this edition.

Two sections describing special programs have been added to Chapters 6 and 15, with a footnote identifying the person who is engaged in the activities described.

The authors and contributors hope that instructors, students, and staff members will enjoy using this edition.

Annie Laurie Crawford
Virginia Curry Kilander

PSYCHIATRIC AND
MENTAL
HEALTH
NURSING EDITION 6

ACKNOWLEDGMENTS

Instructors and students who use the sixth edition will, we believe, like the chapters prepared by four new contributors. They have not only written the chapters bearing their names, but have reviewed, commented, and made helpful suggestions on other chapters.

The authors are especially indebted to the following members of the Eastern State Hospital Staff, Williamsburg, Virginia: Betty Drake, M.S.N., R.N., Nurse Manager, and member of the Nursing Standards Committee; Dorothy Jones, M.S.N., R.N., Clinical Nurse Specialist, Hancock Geriatric Treatment Center; Audrey Waddle, M.S.N., R.N. and Geraldine Coffman, M.S.N., R.N., Nursing Education Department and members of the Nursing Standards Committee; Anne Peet, B.S., R.N., Supervisor, The Therapeutic Community; Alice Richwine, O.T.R., Activities Director, Hancock Geriatric Treatment Center; and Nancy Munnikysen, C.A.V.S., Director Volunteer Services.

Faculty members of the Vocational Schools of Practical Nursing, Lafayette High School, Williamsburg, Virginia and the School of Practical Nursing, Riverside Hospital, Newport News, Virginia have made helpful suggestions.

To some special friends who have encouraged us: Ann Cain, Frances Carter, Cynthia Rector, and Hildegarde Peplau we owe special thanks. Attendance at and participation in "Century Celebration" of 1982 was a powerful stimulus to the preparation of a major revision. We hope this edition also reflects credit on those who have shared generously their knowledge and experiences through the many years of our association. We have learned much from them and the students we have taught.

And finally, to Beth Meisner and Annie Laurie Crawford's niece, Judith Johnson, whose typewriters have stood at "ready" for these past months, many thanks.

Annie Laurie Crawford
Virginia Curry Kilander

CONTRIBUTORS

FAYE GARY HARRIS, Ed.D., R.N., F.A.A.N.
Professor, College of Nursing
University of Florida, Gainesville

JUDITH MORRIS, M.A., R.N., C.S.
Psychiatric Clinical Nurse Specialist
Hampton Veterans Administration Medical Center
Hampton, Virginia

M. TERESA MULLIN, M.S., R.N.
Richmond Services Coordinator
Peninsula Psychiatric Institute,
Hampton, Virginia, and
Adjunct Faculty, Alcohol and Drug Educational Rehabilitation Program
Virginia Commonwealth University
Richmond, Virginia

PATRICIA NOTTINGHAM ROBINSON, M.A., R.N., C.C.N.A.
Director, Clinical Nursing
Peninsula Psychiatric Institute
Hampton, Virginia, and
Visiting Professor
Hampton Institute School of Nursing
Hampton, Virginia

ROBERT VARNADO, M.S.N., R.N.
Instructor, Department of Nursing
McNeese State University
Lake Charles, Louisiana

CONTENTS

CHAPTER 1   *A HISTORICAL PERSPECTIVE*

LEARNING OBJECTIVES

Study of this chapter should prepare the student to:

1. Define mental health.
2. State the early treatment of mentally disordered persons.
3. State why Dorothea Dix and Linda Richards are associated with services to the mentally ill.
4. Identify the aims of the National Mental Health Act.
5. Identify legislation enacted to improve mental health care in your state.
6. Summarize the impact the National Institute of Mental Health has had on the development of psychiatric nursing.
7. State the legal rights of mental patients (see Appendix 1).
8. State some important influences that have contributed to present treatment programs.
9. Identify the special contributions of Hildegarde Peplau and Hattie Bessent to the advancement of psychiatric mental health nursing education and practice.
10. Identify "Century Celebration 1982."

Health is defined by the World Health Organization as a state of complete "mental and physical well-being." The health of an individual is influenced by hereditary traits as well as factors in the environment and the choice of lifestyle.

Mentally healthy persons have been described as those who have developed a mature pattern of problem solving, fulfill their innate capacity for work and for love, are able to cope with crises without assistance beyond the support of family and friends, and whose value system includes wholesome respect for and trust of themselves and others. An individual matter.

Many of the conditions diagnosed as mental disorders are expressed in behavior that is conspicuous, threatening, and disruptive of relationships, or varies significantly from behavior in the society of which the person is a member. Early efforts to cure and control mental disorders included punishment, rejection, abandonment, and compassion.

Early in the 19th century, French and English physicians began to sanction a kindly personal interest in patients by staff members. This was called "Moral Treatment."

The first mentally disordered persons hospitalized in the American colonies were admitted to the Pennsylvania Hospital in Philadelphia. Dr. Benjamin Rush, a signer of the Declaration of Independence, became chief of staff of the Pennsylvania Hospital in 1783. His interest in the mentally ill, the treatment procedures he initiated, and the extensive reports of his work with patients formed the basis for early psychiatric practice in the United States.

The New York Hospital began admitting mentally disordered patients to a basement unit in 1771. The first public hospital for the insane opened in Williamsburg, Virginia in 1773. Two private asylums were established in New England in the early 19th century (McLean Asylum, Waverly, Massachusetts in 1818 and Hartford Retreat, Hartford, Connecticut in 1820). States began building public mental health hospitals in the United States about 1830.

The "moral treatment" practiced in France and England and sanctioned by many early American psychiatrists did not reach all patients in American institutions. In 1841, Dorothea Dix, a Massachusetts schoolteacher, was invited by theology students to teach a Sunday school class to a group of women prisoners. She was appalled and outraged when she found that several mentally ill women were among the prisoners in an overcrowded, unclean, and unheated cell. Putting her teaching career aside, she mounted a lifelong crusade to better the living conditions and treatment for the mentally ill. Her work and influence were felt not only in the United States, but also in Canada, the British Isles, and the European continent.

Dr. John Minson Galt II, a member of the fourth generation of Galts to serve in the management of the insane asylum at Williamsburg, was an eager student of the "moral treatment" being practiced in Europe. Convinced that certain patients could enjoy and profit by living with a family, he proposed that they be sent to live in the community in a supervised setting. He also proposed employing skilled craftsmen to work with and teach patients to become skilled at a craft. These ideas were criticized by a few psychiatrists and ignored by the legislature. In 1858, the *American Journal of Psychiatry* reviewed Dr. Galt's proposals and commented that his long experience should have entitled his ideas to more serious consideration.

NURSING

The first training school for nurses, based on the Nightingale system, was established in 1872 by the New England Hospital for Women and Children. It was here that psychiatric nursing in the United States was developed. Linda Richards, the first nurse to graduate from the one-year course, was instrumental in the establishment of twelve training schools in the United States. Four of these schools were established in mental hospitals because, as she said, ". . . the mentally ill are entitled to as least as good nursing care as the physically ill."

The McLean Asylum, Waverly, Massachusetts, opened the *first training school in a mental hospital in 1882*. Affiliation with Massachusetts General Hospital for instruction in general nursing began in 1886. However, instruction in psychiatric nursing was not included in most of the training schools established by general hospitals. The construction of general hospitals was increasing, but most did not admit psychiatric patients. Linda Richards, with several of the early nursing leaders in the United States, continued to call attention to the importance of training to care for mental patients.

By early 1900, the training of nurses was flourishing in the United States. The Society of Superintendents of Nurses had been formed, and nurses were expressing concern for establishing standards for education and practice.

The first Nurse Practice Act setting state-approved standards for training and authorizing licensure of nurses was passed in 1903. These standards required that students be taught medical, surgical, obstetric, and pediatric

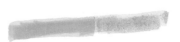

nursing. State and private psychiatric hospitals operating training schools for "mental nurses" were required to arrange affiliation with training schools for instruction in medical, surgical, obstetrics, and pediatrics to qualify the student for licensure as a Registered Nurse. Following their affiliation with a general hospital a few of the nurses selected general nursing practice, but a large number returned to the mental hospitals where they had received their training, or sought employment in other mental hospitals. These were the psychiatric nurses of the early 20th century.

In 1915, the American Nurses Association, with financial support from the National Committee for Mental Hygiene, conducted a study of the 41 training schools in the United States operated by mental hospitals. At this time Linda Richards reiterated her conviction concerning the needs and value of training in psychiatric nursing for all nurses: ". . . a course of study in a state hospital often develops a pupil nurse in an astonishing manner. She must develop a large amount of patience and tact . . . qualities that must be cultivated in nursing the insane."

Isabel Hampton Robb, director of the nursing school, Johns Hopkins Hospital, Baltimore, Maryland, and other nursing leaders continued to promote the need for nursing to focus more attention on the nursing needs of the mentally ill.

The United States' entry into the First World War in 1917 brought sharply into focus the shortage of nurses prepared to work effectively with psychiatric patients. Bloomingdale Hospital, the psychiatric unit of The New York Hospital, is credited with "doing yeoman service" in preparing nurses to work effectively with psychiatric casualties. Smith College conducted intensive short courses for psychiatric aides.

By 1930, collaborative efforts among nursing and psychiatric organizations were increasing. In 1933, Dr. Alfred P. Noyes, speaking to a full session devoted to psychiatric nursing during the National League of Nursing Education Convention, predicted a "bright future for psychiatric nursing."

During the mid 1930s, important developments in the treatment of mental illness (insulin therapy, electrotonic treatment, chemotherapy, psychoanalysis, and advances in psychotherapy) brought new hope for recovery to patients and their families. At that time, 80 percent of hospital beds available for the mentally ill were in state and county hospitals. Five hundred *mental hygiene clinics* had been established and one hundred general hospitals were admitting and treating psychiatric patients.

The entry of the United States into the Second World War in 1941 brought more sharply into focus the need for education in the principles of mental health and psychiatric nursing. Casualties resulting from the hardships and ravages of war placed severe strain on the psychiatric nurse power available for military duty. The number of nursing schools including psychiatric nursing in the basic curriculum increased sharply.

The experiences of the Second World War clearly confirmed the need and desirability of a massive and concerted attack on the cost in human suffering of mental illness. Congress was urged to act by both health professionals and citizens. The first postwar Congress responded by passage of *The National Mental Health Act* in 1946. This act provided for the establishment of the *National Institute of Mental Health* to implement the programs authorized by the Act. The Institute, aware that sufficient numbers of qualified personnel were unavailable to train workers and to staff new community mental health centers, gave first priority to training and to research directed to improving treatment and rehabilitation. Grants were awarded to public and private educational institutions for expansion of educational programs and to individuals for advanced study and research.

Nursing schools moved quickly to expand and to establish additional programs to prepare teachers, supervisors, and researchers.

Congressional and Presidential commissions, legislative acts, regional compacts, state and local laws and ordinances have provided authorization and continue to appropriate funds to support education of all personnel and to expand systems of care, custody, treatment, and prevention.

Hildegarde Peplau's book *Interpersonal Relations in Nursing* published in 1952 had a profound effect on the direction and content of psychiatric/ mental health nursing education and provided a scholarly framework for psychiatric nursing practice and research.

A program directed by Hattie Bessent, and funded by the National Institute of Mental Health, is currently preparing ethnic and racial minority nurses at the doctoral level. These nurses are engaged in education, practice, and research that is adding new dimensions to psychiatric mental health services, especially to America's minority groups.

In November 1982, American nurses convened a gala "Century Celebration" to mark the 100th anniversary of the first formal training in psychiatric nursing in the United States. The progress made during the first century is impressive. Psychiatric nursing is now firmly established as an aspect of all nursing practice and a specialized field of advanced nursing practice. Nurses will continue to increase their leadership in accomplishing the objectives of legislation, community action, and professional practices to assure that the most appropriate therapeutic, rehabilitative, and preventive service is available to each person needing the service. As we enter the second century we can all look back with pride and some humility when we remember those who were truly pioneers, many of whom did not make the history books.

The following brief story of one pioneer career in psychiatric nursing was told to me in the early 1950s by a nurse who was nearing retirement from her position as director of nursing in a large state hospital.

> I went to work as an attendant in the state hospital at sixteen. I was assigned to night duty. We used lanterns to make rounds at night, so all patients were restrained in bed to avoid the possibility one might upset a lantern and set fire to the ward.
>
> When the state hospital opened a training school for nurses I enrolled, graduated, and became a Registered Nurse. During the years, I served as head nurse, supervisor, and finally director of nursing service. I took time out for study twice. The first time I enrolled in a postgraduate course in New York City. Later, when it seemed appropriate for a nurse holding an administrative position to have a degree, I enrolled in a local college and after several years of part-time study obtained a bachelor's degree in sociology.

LEARNING ACTIVITIES

1. Prepare a brief review of the history and current status of the care of the mentally ill in your state. Specify the influence nurses have had on care and treatment.
2. Visit an institution or agency and prepare a report of your observations and any activities you participated in during your visit. Use the form on the next page if allowed by the agency.

BIBLIOGRAPHY

DAIN, N: *Disordered Minds.* Williamsburg in America Series, No VIII. The Colonial Williamsburg Foundation, Williamsburg, 1971.

MANFREDA, M AND KRAMPITZ, S: *Psychiatric Nursing,* ed 10. FA Davis, Philadelphia, 1977.

One Hundred Years of American Psychiatry. Published for the American Psychiatric Association by Columbia University Press, New York, 1944.

PEPLAU, HF: *Interpersonal Relations in Nursing.* GP Putnam's Sons, New York, 1952.

PEPLAU, HF: *Principles of Psychiatric Nursing.* In *American Handbook of Psychiatry.* Basic Books, New York, 1959, pp 1840–56.

```
┌─────────────────────────────────────────────────────────────┐
│               PARTICIPANT OBSERVER ACTIVITIES                 │
│                                                               │
│  Name of institution or agency _____ Date _____ │
│  Main purpose (program) _____  │
│  Activities                                                   │
│                                                               │
│                                                               │
│  Observed                         Participated in             │
│                                                               │
│                                                               │
│  What I learned:                                              │
│                                                               │
│                                                               │
│  Questions I have:                                            │
│                                                               │
│                                                               │
│               Signed: _____  │
└─────────────────────────────────────────────────────────────┘
```

Report of the President's Commission on Mental Health, US Dept of Health and Human Services, Washington, DC, 1980.

ROBERTS, MM: *American Nursing: History and Interpretations.* Macmillan, New York, 1954.

SMOYAK, S AND ROUSLIN, S (EDS): *A Collection of Classics in Psychiatric Nursing Literature.* Charles B Slack, Thorofare, NJ, 1982.

CHAPTER 2　PERSONALITY DEVELOPMENT AND DEFENSE MECHANISMS

LEARNING OBJECTIVES

Study of this chapter should prepare the student to:
1. Define personality.
2. State the influences that generally shape the personality of an individual.
3. List the stages of development of an individual from birth to adulthood.
4. Identify important characteristics associated with each stage of development.
5. List some potential stumbling blocks to progression toward maturity and identify the stage of development at which these stumbling blocks may occur.
6. Define defense mechanisms.
7. Identify and give examples of the use of defense mechanisms at each stage of personality development.

Personality may be defined as the relatively consistent attitudes and behaviors that characterize a person. Development of the personality is influenced by genetic factors and by interactions with the environment that affect a person's personal security, value system, and ability to establish and maintain relationships with others. Normal growth and development depend on the mastery of *psychologic tasks* that increase in complexity as a person moves through stages from the total dependency of the newborn to the independence of a mature and responsible adult.

Knowledge and understanding of personality development are important for nursing personnel. People tend to regress and exhibit behavior characteristic of an earlier stage of development during episodes of physical stress, crises associated with critical illness, and in mental illness. The chairman of the board of a large corporation who is accustomed to directing others and making important decisions daily may, when critically ill, become fearful, dependent, and demanding of special attention. A child who has learned to walk and is toilet trained may, after a brief illness, regress to infancy and require assistance to walk again and re-establish toilet training.

Nurses need to be aware of their own personality development since their responses may either enhance or diminish their effectiveness in working with patients. Family members frequently need support from nurses to cope with the changed behavior of the ill family member. Erickson's Eight Stages of Man are described in terms of developmental tasks. The accomplishment of the previous task prepares the individual for the next one. According to Erickson, the first developmental task confronting a human being is that of acquiring basic trust.

INFANCY (BIRTH TO 1½ YEARS)

An infant is completely dependent on the mother or a mother figure for survival. During this stage, biologic needs (food, shelter, warmth) and psychologic needs (a sense of security that is associated with the provision of food, shelter, and comfort) can be satisfied. For example, sucking is a strong innate reflex by which the infant obtains food, but it also acquires other meanings. The infant whose basic needs are generally satisfied learns trust and develops ability to tolerate the occasional frustration of delay. If response to such basic needs as hunger and comfort is inconsistent or unpredictable, frustration will be reinforced. This may be expressed by angry crying in an effort to evoke a response or by listlessness and apathy. Basic mistrust may be expressed later in aggressive or coercive behavior or by withdrawal, which may interfere with the development of mutually satisfying relationships. The sensory stimulation that occurs as the mother is handling the infant during bathing and feeding allows the infant to learn to differentiate between self and others. By exploring his or her own body and touching others the infant begins to develop a sense of identity and the capacity for independent action begins to emerge. The infant learns to walk, to eat solid foods, and to talk. If speech has developed, "no" may be one of the first words learned.

TODDLER STATE (1½ TO 3 YEARS)

During the toddler stage some satisfaction of a child's instinctual impulses must be given up in response to the demands of others. Toilet training is one of the tasks to be accomplished. A child learns to regulate bowel and bladder functions in a socially acceptable way. If the mother-child relationship facilitates the mother's demand for cleanliness and the child's need to be in command of bodily functions, the child begins to develop a sense of responsibility. Praise for accomplishment teaches the rewards of responsible action and forms the basis for learning to cope with aggressive impulses and modify behavior in accordance with the demands of others. During this stage of development a child also begins to distinguish sexual roles by striving to become like the parent of the same sex. Play, exercise of imagination, and imitation emerge. Girls, for example, delight in "dressing up" in adult clothing—Mother's high-heel pumps are a special attraction.

> *Example:* A young mother and her 3-year-old daughter accompanied a friend to a department store to purchase shoes. As they waited for fitting, the friend noticed the 3-year-old had removed her shoes and was happily tottering around in a pair of high-heel pumps she had taken from a display shelf. When the friend called this to the mother's attention, her amused response was "I'm trying to pretend that she doesn't belong to me." After a brief pause she moved to distract her daughter's attention, retrieved the pumps, and replaced them on the display shelf with an explanation to her daughter. The mother recognized that this was normal behavior so she did not reprimand or embarrass her daughter by making an unpleasant scene; in a friendly discussion she initiated learning respect for the property of others.

EARLY CHILDHOOD (PRESCHOOL)

The early childhood stage is a time of many questions, much curiosity, and fanciful tales. "Why does it rain?" "Where does the rain come from?" "Why does Grandma take her teeth out at night?" "Where does God live?" "I went into the woods and saw a bear with her two children. She told me their names and said I could play with them." "No" is now a favorite word, an expression of the need to establish a personal identity.

Children approaching school age may experience the ambivalence of wanting their mothers to accompany them to school, while looking forward somewhat fearfully to the independence of being a student. If the child has learned that Mother can be trusted, this crisis of early childhood is readily resolved. Talking about school, walking past the school, and planning and selecting school clothes together serve to orient the child to expectations. Many children will have attended nursery or church school, so it can be expected that a child who has these experiences will have achieved a measure of independence.

LATER CHILDHOOD (SCHOOL AGE)

An important step in the later childhood stage of development is that of learning to share, adapting one's own desires and preferences in accordance with others. Energy is channeled into school work and group activities. Friendships are formed with members of the same sex. Members of the opposite sex become targets to be ignored or belittled. Peer-group activity and behavior become important. Compromise in choices of what to do or where to go when leisure time is available is common. An urge to "make something" for a parent, or a group project such as a clubhouse, occurs. Successful completion of a project or task must receive recognition and appreciation from others. During this period, parents nurture a sense of accomplishment by assisting only to the extent that the child indicates help or collaboration is desired. Shared activities with the parent of the same sex nurture a warm and open communication system—important to healthy coping with early adolescent tasks. Acceptance of ethical and moral values is facilitated by an openness that encourages questions and discussions of concerns. Whenever possible, parents enhance a sense of value by setting appropriate limits that communicate a message of worth and trust. Shared secrets among members of one's peer group are common and should be respected by parents and others.

ADOLESCENCE (EARLY AND LATER)

During the early adolescent period, rapid body growth and the emergence of sexual impulses may be disturbing. The struggle to develop a feeling of adequacy and self-confidence frequently causes stress and discomfort. Relationships with family members provide a pattern for resolution of relationships with authority figures. The adolescent must accept more responsibility and show increased independence and maturity. Personality traits that emerge during this stage make up the self-concept of the individual. Many adults tend to look on the exercise of independence at this period of development as rebellion and react negatively to it. However, acting upon one's own perceptions and values at this stage is essential for continuing growth toward maturity. If these values and perceptions are at variance with those of one's parents and result in conflict, communication with parents may diminish. The adolescent may be influenced by peer-group members to defy parents in inappropriate ways. Successful resolution of conflicts is facilitated by verbal communication—a two-way process, where each one talks and each one listens. Parents must be aware that persuasion rather than rigid exercise of authoritarian control is essential. What others in one's peer group are "allowed" to do versus what the parents set as limits must be understood, be realistic, consistent, and accepted. Otherwise, this becomes a source of conflict that may evoke a response of defiance or withdrawal. These interpersonal transactions between parents and adolescents serve to teach the social skills essential for satisfying relationships with peers and with those in authority in society.

Example: The 37-year-old unmarried daughter of a minister described with an extraordinary display of emotion the humiliation she suffered during her teens because she was not allowed to accept invitations to parties unless her younger brother was invited so that he could escort her and bring her home at 9:30 PM. He was then allowed to return to the party. Her mother's explanation was that she must be a model since her father was the local minister. This was in conflict with the mother's expressed disappointment that her daughter was not popular with young men in the church and community.

ADULTHOOD (YOUNG AND MIDDLE YEARS)

During the adulthood stage of development, the potential for intimacy or isolation is paramount. Successful accomplishment of all previous developmental tasks leads to adult maturity. The mature adult enjoys a capacity to do productive work, to express and receive love and esteem, and to maintain self-regulated behavior in society. As the mature young adult approaches the middle years, the rewards of achievement and a comfortable place in society are enjoyed. Guiding the next generation becomes the focus for attention. Interest shifts to concern about adult changes (physical and psychologic), concern for the success of children and the welfare of aging parents.

THE ELDERLY

The ability to enjoy relationships throughout adult and aging years is the outcome of preparation that began and continued with each developmental task. Those who have mastered these tasks continue productivity and social relationships with peers and with members of succeeding generations as they age "gracefully," and accept limits on their independence as this becomes necessary. Some elderly people, no longer able to maintain full independence in their lives, may express objections to change by denial and refusal to accommodate to change or to acknowledge the reality that change is necessary. For many, children become targets of their failure to comply with realistic plans. The defense mechanism of projection is often used to support their resistance to acceptance of their changing status. Others in the retirement years accept physical changes, adjust to retirement, and cope with loss of a spouse and diminished independence.

DEFENSE MECHANISMS

Defense mechanisms are the psychologic processes used by individuals to resolve conflicts and stress that are embarrassing, painful, or threatening. Conflicts and stress may occur within a person, between individuals, or among groups. The defense mechanisms are also used by healthy, well-adjusted people, beginning in early childhood. It is important for parents, teachers, and others to be aware of a child's need to use a defense mechanism, and to allow time for resolution of the conflict, or "cooling off" reaction to the painful or embarrassing experience. If further discussion is indicated, an opportunity for discussion can be delayed until an appropriate time. Many conflicts between marriage partners are resolved by recognition and understanding of the need to use defense mechanisms, or challenged in a hostile manner that further alienates the "defending" partner. Emotionally disturbed and mentally ill persons use defense mechanisms to avoid healthy resolution of conflict. The result is unacceptable behavior. It is important for nurses to be sensitive to a patient's need to use defense mechanisms to cope with a particularly stressful situation. Allowing the patient time to resolve the threat or conflict is essential, and the nurse should not challenge or interfere.

Some of the defense mechanisms used by individuals are discussed in Chapter 3 (Emotional Reactions to Illness and Other Significant Losses). Other defense mechanisms protect and help to manage problems of daily living and threats to one's self-esteem. Definitions and examples of them follow.

Compensation is the substitution of one form of gratification for another that is unavailable or forbidden by circumstances. A young man who is planning a career in athletics, paralyzed in an accident, decides to study law and graduates at the head of his class.

Sublimation allows a person to resolve an urge to unacceptable conduct by substituting socially acceptable behavior. An aggressive person becomes expert in a sport that rewards "rough and tumble" action to win. Another selects a management position where precision is vital, and is rewarded for the quality of the department's performance.

Rationalization is finding a "good reason" instead of admitting the real reason for an act or one's behavior. This is the most commonly used defense mechanism.

Regression is expressed by immature behavior, signaling a return to an earlier stage of development when a person is faced with a painful or threatening situation. During serious illness a person may make unusual demands for attention. The emotionally disturbed person may exhibit behavior that persists over a prolonged period and may be out of proportion to the perceived threat.

Projection is used to deny unacceptable thoughts and feelings by attributing them to another person. This protects the person's self-worth. The patient may claim that a nurse is unfair because the patient has developed a dislike for the nurse. Aggressive mentally ill persons may develop a delusion that someone plans to harm them.

Repression is used to deny or "forget" unpleasant experiences or an embarrassing event. A wife who went to a shopping center "on a quick errand" spent the day shopping for bargains at a sale. When her husband came home from work, she told him that someone parked too close to her car when she finished her errand, so she went back into the store to wait for the car next to hers to be moved and found some real bargains on things they could use. He did not react with anger, but his sense of humor was engaged to finally admit that this was a really unique excuse for an unplanned shopping spree.

Reaction formation is expressed in behavior that is opposite to an unconscious wish. A woman agrees to help with a community project of which she disapproves, but does not wish her friends to know she is opposed to the project.

Displacement is used to substitute an object or a person for another,

Suppression - the process of deliberately forgetting unpleasant thoughts or happenings.

treating the person substituted as if he were the original person or object. One of the classics is the comment about the private "chewed out" by his sergeant who went home and punished his son for a fancied infraction of home rules. The emotionally unstable person may express hatred and act differently toward all authority figures because of experiences with a stern parent.

Dissociation is the blocking out of acutely painful or embarrassing experiences from one's own consciousness.

Fantasy is the use of one's imagination to resolve a problem. A patient may use fantasy as a means of coping with overwhelming problems by retreating from and avoiding reality.

Identification is used when patterning oneself to resemble a person the individual idealizes. A girl in school plans to be a teacher exactly like her favorite teacher. A mentally ill patient feels and acts like a person with whom the patient identifies.

Conversion is a mechanism by which a person translates a psychologic conflict into physical illness. The wife of a prominent physician, brought up in a strict home, attended a woman's college where dancing and card playing were frowned upon. The social group to which she and her husband belonged always held a Saturday night event at which dancing and bridge were entertainment activities. The wife used severe headaches and other forms of illness to avoid attendance until a physician brother-in-law suggested she go to a psychiatric clinic for evaluation. Since her own personal scruples were not a barrier, she willingly took dancing and bridge lessons in secret to surprise and delight her husband with her new skills. Several counseling sessions had helped her to understand the probable source of her "headaches."

LEARNING ACTIVITIES

1. Think of three or more experiences you consider to have influenced your personality development. Prepare a "memory sketch" and study the content to assess your interactions with peers, supervisors, members of your family, and friends.
2. Select a patient for study. Review the patient's personal history and identify clues to interactions with a mother or another person during three of the developmental stages. Plan, with your instructor, to interview the patient. Request the patient's permission to record the interview. Focus the interview and record the responses to questions on the patient's interpretation of the interactions you have selected. Does the patient

believe that childhood experiences relate to the present problems? Identify the therapeutic approaches you will use in working with this patient. Use the nursing process. Prepare a report of your work with the patient, stating the degree of achievement of the goals the patient and you establish.

3. Select several patients with whom you work who show pronounced use of defense mechanisms. Plan a team conference for discussion of the use of these defense mechanisms by patients. Discuss the behavior displayed and the way this behavior is contributing to the patient's problems. Plan with your co-workers some strategies for helping the patient gain insight and change behavior.
4. Patient identification with members of the staff may be an important aspect of treatment. Discuss the kinds of identification that are to be encouraged, discouraged, and the ways you might accomplish this.
5. Identify the defense mechanisms you are most likely to use to deal with stress, threats, or disappointments. (This is for your personal study, to discuss only if you wish.)

BIBLIOGRAPHY

ANDERSON, BG: *The Aging Game.* McGraw-Hill, New York, 1981.

BABCOCK, DE: *Introduction to Growth, Development and Family Life,* ed 3. FA Davis, Philadelphia, 1972.

CARTER, FM: *Psychosocial Nursing,* ed 3. Macmillan, New York, 1981.

ERICKSON, E: *Childhood and Society.* WW Norton, New York, 1964.

ERICKSON, E: *Youth and Crisis.* WW Norton, New York, 1968.

MASLOW, AH: *Toward a Psychology of Being,* ed 3. Van Nostrand Reinhold, New York, 1968.

PETERSON, MH: *Understanding defense mechanisms.* Am J Nurs 71:1651–1674, 1972.

Denial - Denying feelings or thoughts.

Fixation - Getting stuck in enviroment

Coping — specific acts to deal c̄ stress, difficulties
c̄ over use of defense mechanisms.

CHAPTER 3   EMOTIONAL REACTIONS TO ILLNESS AND OTHER SIGNIFICANT LOSSES

LEARNING OBJECTIVES

Study of this chapter should prepare the student to:
1. State the factors that influence an individual's reaction to illness and other losses.
2. Identify defense mechanisms frequently used by ill persons to cope with illness and other losses.
3. Identify some barriers to healthy coping with illness.
4. Discuss dependency needs of a patient.
5. Describe the health-promoting activities nurses use to assist a patient and family to cope with illness and loss.
6. Identify and describe support services available to patients in your community.

Illness is a threatening experience, causing anxiety which disrupts emotional stability. Illnesses and injuries that produce the highest degree of threat are those which involve loss of significant aspects of the self, such as loss of body function and/or parts, loss of mobility and/or independence, and threatened loss of life. Symptoms of brain impairment, such as disorientation, confusion, hallucinations, and loss of memory are also serious threats to patients and their families.

The level of anxiety experienced by the patient may be influenced by family beliefs and attitudes about the cause and the expected outcome of the particular condition. The personality of the patient also influences the degree of threat the illness poses. A person who has developed an optimistic view or who generally copes with crises in a mature manner will experience the disruption in emotional stability, but to a lesser degree than one who views even minor illness as a catastrophe. The anxiety of the patient may be reinforced by the anxiety expressed by the family.

DENIAL

Denial may be the initial response to an illness or accident which the patient perceives as especially threatening to plans for future activities, economic security, or family stability. This is a psychologic *defense mechanism* that temporarily protects the patient from the full impact of the illness. Denial may be used by members of the patient's family until they are psychologically ready to cope with the change in the health of the person who is ill, and possibly with the inevitable changes in the family lifestyle or relationships.

Many patients use partial denial and participate in their treatment plans while seeming to deny the seriousness of the illness. For others, the denial is so complete it interferes with treatment.

The patient with a life-threatening illness or the victim of an accident that also involves loss of body parts or functions may use varying degrees of denial ranging from feeling that "this isn't really happening to me" even though there is awareness that it is.

Example: The patient who received a diagnosis of breast cancer may say, "This is not really cancer, only a small tumor." If the cancer is untreatable and there is serious discomfort and vomiting, the patient may attribute such symptoms to tests, although the tests were made several weeks earlier.

Example: The young man who has received a head injury in an accident and who appears conscious, but cannot answer questions about the accident, may say, "I was asleep when it happened, so I don't have any idea."

Example: The airline pilot who has suffered a severe heart attack denies the inability to return to work after there has been time for sufficient rest and recovery.

A strong need for the self-protection provided by the use of denial may cause patients forced with major changes in career, lifestyle, or even a threat to life, to hear only what they wish to hear, or to deny that there has been any discussion of the prognosis.

Denial is a protective mechanism that automatically limits the amount of information the patient and/or family must cope with when unable to face the overwhelming threat of the illness all at once. The full significance of the illness becomes real gradually.

ANGER

Anger is a common reaction to anxiety associated with injury or illness which is most likely to result in disfigurement or disability. The patient feels frustrated, fearful, and helpless. The threat to one's sense of wholeness increases anxiety, which can readily be expressed through anger. The patient's feelings of anger and frustration are also usually shared by family members.

The anger may be directed toward nursing personnel, the hospital, or the physician. It may be expressed by excessive demands for attention.

Example: A 22-year-old man received a spinal injury in a skiing accident. His legs were paralyzed. His family complained that his doctor did not give him proper attention, although the doctor saw him daily. He also kept his call light on almost constantly. His demands had to do with adjustments of the window or shade, rarely about his needs or physical comfort.

Feelings of anger are more comfortable than acute anxiety. Anger is considered a healthier reaction than indifference, apathy, or withdrawal, all of which reflect a feeling of hopelessness and readiness to give up.

The potential for health is inherent in the forces within the personality that constantly work toward emotional equilibrium when the self is threatened. During a major illness the forces that maintain balance are weakened, and the level of anxiety is increased. At this time the patient is likely to react with regression and increased dependency.

REGRESSION

Regression is a common adaptive defense mechanism to illness. The *regression* permits the person to return unconsciously to less mature behavior, thus reducing the level of anxiety and permitting rest and the use of diminished energy for healing and recovery. Regression makes it possible for the patient to tolerate the loss of independence and adopt the "passive patient" role during the illness. As a temporary behavior, regression is useful to help patients adapt during the serious stages of their illness. Interests and concerns are directed to self: this is commonly referred to as egocentric behavior.

Example: The voice of a 55-year-old president of a trucking company in the intensive care unit with a heart attack sounds childlike when he requests something. He also lies in the fetal position when his wife visits.

At this stage in the patient's illness, nursing personnel who understand this reaction recognize that the patient has the right to be sick and to behave in a self-centered manner. They can respond to the patient's concern with warm, caring, accepting, and nonjudgmental attention, accepting the patient's behavior. The patient needs to feel safe, respected, and cared for. The ill person feels keenly the loneliness and separation from normal daily activities. The hospital environment and unfamiliar equipment and procedures contribute to increased fears. Concern about the expectations of health personnel is frequently a cause for anxiety. "What will happen to me if I do not behave as a good patient should?" suggests the stance of a 3-year-old not yet secure about parental expectations. The anxiety of the patient may also be reinforced by family members who approach nursing personnel, seeking information or special services for the patient. If nursing personnel see this as unwarranted interference and show disapproval in their responses, the patient may feel trapped between family anxiety for his or her welfare, and the nurse's view of the behavior as interference.

Dependency needs of patients during serious illnesses allow nursing personnel to provide comfort, security, and attention consistent with recognition that the patient has a right to self-centered behavior during a certain stage of illness. Understanding that regression and dependency are normal in serious illness helps the nurse to deal with them appropriately.

Throughout life there is a drive toward independence, which at times is in conflict with the remembered comfort, warmth, and security of having dependency needs satisfied during infancy and childhood. The peak of the push toward independence occurs during the toddler and adolescent periods. A person who is able to grow in independence while having dependency needs met without undue pressure is likely to develop into one who is able to function satisfactorily in adult roles. Healthy adult roles require a balance of independence, dependence, and interdependence. Such a person is capable of experiencing satisfaction from both giving and receiving.

ALTERATIONS IN INDEPENDENCE-DEPENDENCE

The independence-dependence balance is threatened by illness as a person faces the realization that many accustomed activities are restricted. The airline pilot hospitalized in an intensive care unit by a serious coronary attack experiences the helplessness of infancy. Since this person has resolved the independence-dependence conflict, tolerating the dependence of critical illness is acceptable until there is no longer the need to accept dependence. For such a person encouragement by the nurse to move toward regaining independence as recovery progresses is natural, expected, and welcome. Patients need to feel that they have some control over what is happening to them. One of the earliest experiences toward regaining independence may be the patient's participation in planning care and treatment schedules. If the illness is expected to alter the lifestyle, require preparation for a different career choice, and restrict previously planned activities, the patient may express anxious feelings concerning the future and seek information during convalescence that will be useful in dealing with the problems the expected change presents.

Example: A woman with a colostomy appeared to listen intently to instructions given by the nurse in preparation for her discharge from the hospital. Only a few questions were asked, however, and the patient appeared to assure the nurse that she felt she could cope with her situation at home. She had even expressed confidence that she could return to work promptly. The day following the discharge she called the nurse at the hospital, and in a near panic implored the nurse to come to her home to help her. The nurse went at once to the patient's house to find her in tears and convinced that she would never be able to return to work or normal social relationships. The nurse became aware that the patient's anxiety resulted because her equipment and her bathroom were not like those at the hospital, and she believed she had forgotten some of the steps in the care procedure. The nurse went to her home daily for one week, as she each day encouraged her to gradually handle the situation. At the end of the week, the patient was pleased with her own competence and said, "I can now return to work without fear of embarrassment."

GRIEF

Grief is the term used to identify the feelings and reactions that normally follow a loss of great significance to a person. There are many kinds of losses. Those related to health may involve a loss of body part or function and/or disfigurement. Some losses are related to self-esteem, pride, and independence. Others may be related to job, status, or financial security. The most profound losses are often related to the loss of a loved one, either through death or separation, or the impending loss of one's own life. Individuals vary in their reactions, depending on the meaning of the loss in their personal lives, their strength of personality, and flexibility, and the support available from family and friends. Increasing attention is being focused on the meaning and need for support to the elderly who are faced with the loss of family or significant others.

The process of grieving involves *adaptation to loss*. This is essential to healthy adjustment and follows a pattern of behavior that includes:

Sadness and depression. How will I manage? What do I have left to live for?
Anxiety. I must sell my house and go to live among strangers. I can't live here alone.
Anger. Why did this happen to me? Why couldn't I have gone first?
Guilt. Maybe I could have done more, made him see a doctor sooner or more often.
Helplessness. What am I to do?
Loneliness. I manage during the day when I am busy, but I can hardly stand the nights alone.
Fear. What will I do if a burglar breaks in? What will happen to me if I get sick here all alone?

Some of these expressions are common to the death of a spouse, the breakup of a family by divorce or separation, and some to parents who lose a child. Some degree of denial and ambivalence are common to the grief experience. Unresolved grief has the potential for the development of both physical and mental health problems.

Grieving persons need to express their feelings to interested, accepting persons. They need to understand that the feelings they are experiencing are a normal and necessary part of the process of learning to live with loss. Support of family, friends, and of health personnel are important factors in the adaptation of an individual who has sustained a loss. Members of the family and friends of a person grieving over a loss also need support and understanding, as well as an opportunity to share their feelings. Nursing personnel may need to initiate a conversation that lets the person know that the grief is natural and that health workers are available to help one understand and to help. Many self-help and sharing groups are sponsored by churches and volunteer organizations, as well as by neighborhoods.

ALTERATIONS IN BODY IMAGE

The body image is an integral part of the self-concept, which includes the feelings and the internal picture an individual carries about his or her body and self. The loss of a part of the body or major body function causes a change in body image. Certain areas and functions have special meaning to an individual — the face, head, genitals, and breasts are invested with considerable emotional significance. When any of these parts of the body are damaged or removed, the individual is likely to react with increased anxiety, denial, anger, and depression. Adaptation to these losses is affected by a number of factors. Change that comes on gradually is less threatening than a sudden and unexpected change that may be the result of an accident. External changes frequently produce greater anxiety than internal changes. The support available to a patient and family is crucial to healthy adjustment, and everyone should be encouraged to express their feelings about the change that has taken place. Information and instructions which recognize the importance of their concerns, and help them to anticipate and deal with problems associated with the change, will assist with the necessary adjustments.

Working through feelings is a gradual process. Intellectual acceptance of the change occurs before emotional adjustment is achieved. Even when a patient understands and accepts the facts of change, it takes longer to integrate the loss into an individual's self-image and to resolve the anger and depression associated with it. The grieving process the patient experiences is necessary for healthy adaptation to significant body alterations. If the patient and family realize that these feelings and reactions are normal and temporary, they will be less frightened and can look forward to a return to emotional stability. The patient's ability to look at and talk about the changed part of the body are early indications that he or she is beginning to deal realistically with the situation.

Support groups, composed of persons who have experienced similar loss, or sponsored by health agencies and community organizations, are also prepared to help. One of these groups, Reach to Recovery, of the American Cancer Society, is composed of members who have had breast cancer surgery. The members visit patients in hospitals and their homes to help in adapting following such surgery.

Patient's Symptoms and Behavior	Suggested Nursing Interventions
Changes in sleep pattern, difficulty falling asleep and early awakening.	Change in sleep habits is a common reaction to anxiety.

General restlessness, vague unpleasant feeling of apprehension.

Anxiety. Guidance in advance of changes involves talking about the change and some of the reactions and problems patient may have to deal with.

Conscious avoidance of considering the possibility of serious disabling illness.

Suppression. Anxiety is uncomfortable and avoided if possible.

Read extensively on the incidence and prognosis of breast cancer.

Planned activities to keep busy and involved.

Tries to maintain control by knowing and intellectualizing.

Activity reduces anxiety.

First postoperative day felt numb, could not believe reality of surgery; felt buffeted about by the forces of life.

Felt comforted and cared for when nurse washed face and helped brush teeth.

Nursing care focuses on safety, security, comfort, and caring. Meeting physical needs with concern communicates acceptance.

Acceptance of dependent state.

When assisted to bathroom with accompanying tubes and bottles felt sudden, violent anger at the indignity and helplessness of the situation.

Feelings of helplessness and dependency create anxiety; high anxiety leads to anger. Dependency may be very threatening to an individual accustomed to being in control. Encourage participation in care where possible, give choices to alleviate feelings of helplessness.

Could not look at incision on 1st postoperative day. Carefully watched and listened to doctor and nurse as dressing was changed. Promised to look the 2nd day.

How others react influences how the patient feels about the altered part. Looking at incision is an early step toward adaptation. Nurse should be aware and in control of her own reaction to the incision.

Sleeplessness, restlessness, pacing.

Anxiety. Encourage sharing of thoughts and feelings; encourage walking and activity.

Talked readily with family and friends about the surgery. Patient felt as if talk was not about self but about some other person.

Beginning acknowledgement; depersonalization. Talking about the surgery is an early step in adapting to change.

Felt mutilated and ugly. Raged and cried.

Provide acceptance and support. Encourage femininity and attractive grooming; realistic praise for aspects of femininity that exist.

Increased crying first with family and close friends; later cried with nurses.

Provide privacy; show support. Crying is a healthy release of feelings.

Angry feelings toward the surgeon; "Why did he remove the entire

Encourage expression of thoughts and feelings. Do not react to anger with breast when the cancer was so small?"

Bitter complaints about the terrible food served.

Why didn't this happen to someone else? Feelings of aloneness and isolation.

Felt anger when packing to go home.

Prayed for complete recovery; promised God if she had another chance she would be a better Christian.

Felt vulnerable; could be pushed over with a feather; felt like a "wet noodle."

Felt depressed. Periodically overwhelmed by unexpected short crying spells. Crying and depression gradually subside.

Felt self as different and impaired; attention focused on lost or damaged part. At home felt some shame with friends. "What will they think of me?"

Gradually ceased identifying self with lost part and began to feel normal.

Thankful for recovery; it could have been worse. Thankful for all that remains. Good feelings about self; pleased with the ability to live through the experience and be stronger for it.

anger. Listen and show understanding.

Displacement. Anger gives feelings of power; replaces anxiety and helplessness. Show willingness to try to provide food liked by patient.

Anger. Encourage ventilation of feelings and reassure these are normal and will pass with time. Warmth, concern, and interested help overcome the isolation of serious illness.

Anger displaced.

Bargaining for life. Reaching for spiritual support; suggest chaplain visit.

Postoperative fatigue and emotional vulnerability. Be supportive; assist with activities patient finds difficult.

Grief. Listen; accept crying as healthy. Encourage feelings. Provide information, show willingness to help and do what is possible.

It is more acceptable to be different in the hospital than it is away from the hospital.

Time with support is important in adaptation. Breasts, prostheses such as colostomy bag, lost limbs loom large as part of identity.

Adaptation; resolution of feelings, acceptance, self-esteem.

LEARNING ACTIVITIES

The challenge to nursing personnel who witness and share the emotional impact on the patient posed by serious illness and catastrophic accidents that leave physical and emotional scars requires sensitivity, compassion, and a realistic optimism to assist the patient to emerge with ego strength equal to the task of adaptation.

1. Review the studies of individual reactions to illness that posed a poten-

tial threat to life and a certainty of change in body image. Both of these threats are increasingly common in the population.

2. Assume or recall that you or a member of your family has received a diagnosis which poses a threat to health, security, or physical wholeness. Prepare a report that describes your reactions and behavior. Summarize the actions which you consider to have been positive and/or negative.

3. Select a support service agency and request an appointment to visit and learn about the services offered. Prepare to report your findings in a class session, describing how you will use this information with your patients. (Each student should, if possible, select a different agency, including both official and voluntary agencies—see Appendix 2).

BIBLIOGRAPHY

Anxiety, recognition and intervention (programmed instruction). Am J Nurs 65:127, 1965.

CARTER, FM: *Psychosocial Nursing,* ed 3. Macmillan, New York, 1981.

ENGEL, GL: *Grief and grieving.* Am J Nurs 64:93, September, 1964.

FRANCES, GM AND MUNJAS, B: *Promoting Psychological Comfort.* William C Brown, Dubuque, 1975.

PEPLAU, HF: *Interpersonal Relations in Nursing.* GP Putnam's Sons, New York, 1952.

PETERSON, MH: *Understanding defense mechanisms.* Am J Nurs 72:1651–1674, 1972.

ROBINSON, L: *Psychological Aspects of the Care of Hospitalized Patients,* ed 3. FA Davis, Philadelphia, 1979.

SAXTON, D AND HARING, PW: *Care of Patients with Emotional Problems,* ed 3. CV Mosby, St Louis, 1979.

CHAPTER 4   # THE BRIEF PSYCHIATRIC EXAMINATION*

Faye Gary Harris, Ed.D., R.N.

The psychiatric assessment is like no other type of health care assessment. The nurse, from the moment of initial contact, begins to "size up" the patient. Personal/intimate information is solicited during the interview process. Although sensitivities, manifestations, conflicts, and perceptions of the self are components that the therapist possesses, the nurse is expected to learn to understand and control personal thoughts and feelings and assess the data from an objective point of view. A structured-type assessment guide might be helpful for assessments in both inpatient and outpatient situations.

ASSESSMENT GUIDE

  I. Vital statistics
    A. Name.
    B. Address and phone number.

---

*The brief psychiatric examination is performed by a psychiatric or other mental health professional in private practice, or by a member of the professional staff of an institution or agency. The findings of the examination form the basis of the treatment program for the patient. Understanding the basis for the treatment plan assists staff members to work more effectively with the patient.

C. Date of birth, age, and sex.
D. Highest education attained, employment if appropriate, parents' occupations.
E. Closest friend or relative.
F. Name and relationship of person who accompanied patient to interview.

II. What is the chief complaint?
   A. How long has the problem existed?
   B. What was the patient's thinking at time decision was made to seek help?

III. Identification of the present illnesses
   A. What physical/mental problems has patient experienced? How long? Describe the treatment received. List operations and reasons for intervention and fluctuations in weight patterns.
   B. List all medications that patient has taken—prescribed and/or non-prescribed.
      1. Alcohol.
      2. Over-the-counter drugs.
      3. Birth control drugs.
      4. Street drugs—marijuana, LSD, etc.
      5. A mixture of street drugs and alcohol.
      6. Were seizures associated with drug experiences? This area is of particular importance when patient is prepubertal or pubertal (adolescent).

IV. Appearance
   The appearance of each family member should be recorded. Include:
      1. Dress.
      2. Mood.
      3. Conformity/nonconformity to social class mores.

V. Pervasive affect
   A. Capture attitudes about the illness/the patient.
   B. Be cautious for feelings of hostility, anger, or resentment toward the interviewer, other family members, or the identified patient.

VI. Motor, thought, and speech patterns
   A. Observe all physical activities, such as:
      1. Nail biting.
      2. Restlessness.
      3. Sweating palms.
      4. Irritability.
   B. Observe the nature of coordination of eye-hand movements.

C. Observe gross motor activities, e.g., walking, skipping/walking/talking simultaneously.

D. Identify predominate themes in conversation.

E. Record usage of specific words.

F. Watch for fragmented speech.

G. Can patient make a point without extraneous materials?

H. Can patient make eye contact without difficulty?

I. Are neologisms present in the content?

J. Does the affect fit with the topics being discussed? (Does sad content elicit sad affect?)

K. Is the patient suspicious? If so, about what? Who are the significant others?

L. Record the rate of speech, pitch, and the difficulty/lack of difficulty in communication.

M. Observe and record the therapist's overall impression of this area.

N. Ask patient if thoughts of suicide have ever been entertained. If so, when? What were the circumstances? How were these thoughts controlled? *Would suicide still be an option?*

O. Observe for obsessions (a persistent thought or feeling that defies logic and is uncomfortable and non-goal-directed for the patient).

P. Observe for perseveration (repetitious thoughts and actions that occur because patient cannot make shifts of thoughts and/or motor responses smoothly).

Q. Ask patient to relate recurrent dreams and/or dreams considered to be of significance.

R. Ask patient to describe daydreams that might be recurrent.

S. Identify the feelings and perceptions the patient has about self, specifically:

    1. Like what parent/person?

    2. Ugly or pretty, dumb or smart, etc?

    3. What will the future be like? What and who makes the future like that?

VII. Abnormal perception and memory

A. Assess for hallucination (false perceptions that occur without any stimulation from the external environment; these might occur because of drug usage, medications, loss of sleep, extreme stress, and/or functional psychosis*), which might be:

    1. Tactile—touch.

---

*Functional psychosis implies no organic basis for a disorder.

      2. Formication—feeling that something is crawling under the skin.

      3. Kinesthetic—position and movement.

      4. Lilliputian—perceptions that people are tiny creatures.

      5. Auditory—hearing voices.

      6. Gustatory—taste.

      7. Olfactory—smell.

      8. Visual—sight.

   B. Can patient remember past events accurately?

   C. Can patient recall recent events accurately?

   D. Does patient practice a "selective loss" of certain events and feelings?

   E. Observe for confabulation, in which patient pieces in memory losses with content that is not true.

VIII. Make a general summary statement about the patient, including general impressions and areas of difficulties experienced by the interviewer.

  IX. A differential assessment for organic brain syndrome (OBS) must be considered. Frequently, the functional psychosis manifests the same types of symptoms that clinicians find in OBS. The common symptoms which one must be able to recognize include:

   A. Memory impairment

      1. Observe for:

        a. Forgetting current events.

        b. Possible memory of past events with some accuracy.

      2. The assessment of memory impairments must occur after the symptoms of functional psychosis and neurosis have been determined and treated.

   B. Disturbance in orientation

      1. Determine whether the patient can remember time sequence, events that occur in sequence.

      2. Assess for orientation to time, place, and person.

        a. Time. Ask:

          1) What is today?

          2) What month is it?

          3) What year is this?

          4) Name a significant current event that recently happened.

        b. Place. Ask: Where are you now?

    c. Person. Who the patient is. Ask for some evidence, such as:
       1) What do you do for a living?
       2) Where do you live?

C. Deficient judgment

This is a most difficult area to discern. The clinician can evaluate how a person might think concerning consequences of a given behavior or situation. The consequences must be evaluated in the appropriate cultural context of the patient. Ask:

1. Do you consider comments that others make about you?
2. Are you good at "sizing up" people? What do you do with this information?
3. Do you like to take chances? Give some examples.

D. Defect in intellect

The clinician needs a baseline knowledge about the patient's vocabulary, word usage, sentence structure, and vocational and avocational interests.

1. Ask patient to add, subtract, and multiply.
2. Discuss content that patient is familiar with and observe for:
    a. Word associations.
    b. Sentence structuring.
    c. Conclusive statements.
3. Use the patient's work habits and environs as data from which observations can be made.
4. Determine whether the current word usage, information processing, and conclusive statements being made by the patient are characteristic, low, or high functioning for the patient.

E. Altered affect

The affect change can be gradual or abrupt. Family members and clinicians observe that:

1. The patient might easily become extremely aggravated.
2. Components of the same situation may cause laughter and, seconds later, crying.
3. A no reaction to any stimulus can be noticed, too. Here the patient just does not respond to sorrow, humor, intimacy, etc.

Other pathologic adaptive responses might occur in later stages of the OBS, e.g., a suspicious-type person may become extremely paranoid and dangerous. These exaggerated forms of responses may be perplexing to family members who never experienced these characteristics in relation to their loved one before.

BIBLIOGRAPHY

BOCKAR, J: *Primer for the Nonmedical Psychotherapist.* Spectrum Publications, New York, 1976.

HARRIS, FG AND WILSON, L: *Mental health problems in children—Assessment.* In SNIDER, J (ED): *Handbook of Clinical Nursing.* McGraw-Hill, New York, 1979.

NICHOLI, AM: *History and mental status.* In NICHOLI, AM (ED): *The Harvard Guide to Modern Psychiatry.* The Belknap Press, Cambridge, 1978.

NICHOLI, AM: *The Therapist-patient relationship.* In NICHOLI, AM (ED): *The Harvard Guide to Modern Psychiatry.* The Belknap Press, Cambridge, 1978.

SIMMONS, J: *The Psychiatric Examination of Children.* Lea & Febiger, Philadelphia, 1976.

CHAPTER 5   *COMMUNICATIONS*

LEARNING OBJECTIVES

> *Study of this chapter should prepare the student to:*
> 1. Define communication.
> 2. Identify the various forms of communication.
> 3. State the bases for therapeutic communication and give examples.
> 4. Describe the use and influence of the different forms of public information.

Communication is a universal aspect of human behavior with the purpose of transmitting information to and receiving information from others. *Webster's New International Dictionary* states that messages are given and received through "talk, gestures, symbols and writing, etc."

Verbal communication (talk) includes face-to-face conversation between persons. Messages received by radio, television, lectures to groups, and entertainment in song and theater are also verbal forms of communication. Nurses use verbal communication to praise achievement, to talk with patients, to share information with families of patients and staff members, and to instruct students.

Nonverbal communication makes use of gestures, symbols, writing, and pictures to inform, instruct, comfort, or repel. A facial expression coupled with a gesture can convey a variety of positive and negative messages: joy, friendship, welcome, and — the most meaningful of all to an infant or young child — the message of love, security, and understanding. Anger, contempt, and disgust are clearly signaled by facial expressions. A gesture may have a certain meaning to one person or group and an entirely different meaning to another person or group. Written words have no value if the person to whom they are addressed is not familiar with the language in which the message is written. Even in a familiar language, messages should be written to convey the meaning of the message to both the sender and the receiver. A symbol may confuse and serve as a source of anxiety or even danger to a person if the meaning of the symbol is unknown to the recipient.

THERAPEUTIC COMMUNICATION

The phrase "therapeutic communication" is frequently used in psychiatric/ mental health nursing practice. What does it mean? For purposes of this discussion we can place definitions of the two words together to readily understand the concept. Communication was just defined; *therapeutic* is defined in *Webster's New World Dictionary* as "to nurse; curative."

In communications with patients, nursing personnel have as their primary goal the establishment of a therapeutic relationship. In simpler terms, the nurse directs communication toward work with the patient to identify the current or potential health problem; to examine the resources available and the potential for coping; to plan, and to implement and evaluate on a continuing basis the results of the action taken. This may not be a "cure" in the traditional sense, but a utilization of resources to achieve a defined goal.

The bases for therapeutic communication are sensitivity and trust. *Sensitivity* implies an ability to listen and observe, to assure that the patient feels free to speak without interruption and without a salvo of advice or questions, both of which may serve as barriers to therapeutic communication.

A *trusting relationship* between nurse and patient is facilitated by complete and accurate information which is relevant to the patient's felt needs as well as comfort and security. Most patients are anxious or fearful and often confused by details of admission procedures, especially if there has been no previous hospitalization. The staff member who is sensitive to that anxiety will welcome and escort the patient in an unhurried manner to the appropriate unit, and make introductions to other patients and staff. Much of the orientation information needed by patients may be posted on unit bulletin boards, or presented to them in printed form. Nursing personnel should show patients the bulletin board, review the information, and tell patients they are free to seek explanations of information that is not understood. Written communication implies that the staff considers patients competent to use the information appropriately. Nursing personnel should be alert and sensitive to the need for clarification and reassurance to confused, depressed, and withdrawn patients. Remind patients that nursing personnel are on duty around the clock and can get in touch with physicians and other staff members if questions involve them.

Some basic concepts of therapeutic interpersonal communication have been identified by psychiatric/mental health nurses and are relevant to all nursing practice.

Nurses must understand how their own behavior influences their interactions with others. The nurse must be aware of how her responses and the nonverbal expressions of her feelings inhibit or facilitate a therapeutic relationship. A response to an anxious patient, "I must finish this task so I cannot talk with you now," should be followed by, "but I will talk with you in half an hour. I appreciate your willingness to wait." Keep the promise to return in half an hour. This facilitates trust and assures the patient of your concern.

Both the nurse and the patient bring *expectations of self and of each other* to the nurse-patient relationship. Acceptance of and respect for differences in beliefs, variations in lifestyle, and ethnic and racial traditions and values are important to therapeutic relationships. Within the framework of acceptance and respect, there is also the concept that the nurse has a responsibility to promote and assist in developing a healthy lifestyle.

Mental health staff members use the collaborative process to assess with patients their assets, strengths, and goals as a basis for realistic planning. The treatment method selected for the patient may influence communication among staff members and between staff members and patients. The treatment plan must be understood by nursing personnel for appropriate response to questions and comments by patients.

If the treatment plan assumes that continuity of service will be advised to or sought by the patient when discharged, it may be appropriate to involve a representative of the service agency, a family member, or an individual or group selected by the patient in the discharge planning. A list of community service and volunteer groups can be found in Appendix 2. Members of these groups offer various support services to families of chronically ill persons who wish to continue caring for the chronically ill member. Support services may also be recommended for patients who will live in group homes or self-care facilities. If the idea of support services is new to the patient or family, the list may be helpful in making a selection.

Public hospitals discharging patients to boarding homes plan visits by the patient to several homes so patients may make their own choice. The patient is usually accompanied on the visit by a social worker and a nurse.

Many nursing homes provide transportation and day care for patients suffering from Alzheimer's disease, Huntington's chorea, Parkinson's disease, and other conditions of the elderly. For families all of whose members work, this type of "day care" provides safety for the patient. In many instances, the stimulus of others in the environment, a nutritious meal at noon, and a planned program of activities usually slow the debilitating effect of isolation.

PUBLIC INFORMATION AND NURSING

There is a continuing flow of information concerning mental health which includes personal health practices and available health services from all forms of communication media. Written work may be found in newspapers, magazines, brochures, announcements of special lectures, workshops, and health center programs. Television announcements, docudramas, and documentaries of personal experience convey information. Computers and satellites will be used more extensively to gather and transmit information. Tape-recorded reports to incoming teams of nursing personnel report patients' conditions and any special needs or problems on the hospital unit. Television monitors from a central station keep nurses informed about patients' vital signs, and provide two-way talk between nurses on the station and the patient in the room. Teleconference, a conference by telephone for a number of participants, makes possible transmission of information between a university center and rural health workers, allowing many more staff members from a unit to participate in continuing education programs to update their knowledge. The extent of communication among mental health personnel seems unlimited.

These developments have three important implications for nursing practice: (1) the widespread development and use of machines must not replace the human aspects (the art of nursing), (2) the responsibility of keeping informed to respond appropriately to patients' questions and misunderstandings about what they have seen or heard, and (3) the responsibility to take action when nurses are portrayed in an inappropriate manner or ignored altogether in public information about providers of mental health services.

> *Example:* A recent edition of a nationally distributed publication devoted several pages to a description of mental health services. Nurses and nursing were not mentioned, yet the number of registered nurses employed in mental health and psychiatric nursing services far outnumbers those from two other professions whose services were reported in detail. Nurses have an obligation to their profession in such instances to speak out in the interest of the public they serve.

Katherine Steele's second textbook on psychiatric nursing was published in 1936 with the recommendation that it be read by patients' families. The author was keenly aware of the value of improving communication between the patient and significant others.

LEARNING ACTIVITIES

1. Prepare a report of your communication with a patient; describe the patient's response and your assessment of the effectiveness of the communication.
2. Request your instructor's assistance in preparing a nursing care plan for a patient, using a specific example of the patient's condition. Use the nursing process. Identify examples of therapeutic communication, using quotes, and list any barriers that occurred.
3. If possible, participate in a plan for a patient who is being referred to a service agency.

BIBLIOGRAPHY

BAILEY, DS AND DREYER, SO: *Therapeutic Approaches to the Care of the Mentally Ill.* FA Davis, Philadelphia, 1977.

CARTER, FM: *Psychosocial Nursing,* ed 3. Macmillan, New York, 1981.

FLAGG, JM: *Consultation in community residences for the chronically Ill.* Psychosoc Nurs Ment Health Serv vol 20 (no 12):30–35, 1982.

LEWIS, GK: *Nurse-Patient Communication,* ed 2. William C Brown, Dubuque, 1973.

SMOYAK, SA AND ROUSLIN, S (EDS): *A Collection of Classics in Psychiatric Nursing Literature.* Charles B Slack, Thorofare, NJ, 1982.

CHAPTER 6   *TREATMENT METHODS*

Robert Varnado, M.S.N., R.N.

LEARNING OBJECTIVES

Study of this chapter should prepare the student to:
1. Describe the types of psychotherapeutic treatments discussed in this chapter.
2. Identify the goals of the various treatments.
3. Identify the classifications of psychopharmacological agents used in treatment in combination with psychotherapeutic methods.
4. List conditions for which certain drugs are prescribed.
5. Describe the nursing observations and appropriate actions associated with reactions to the drugs.
6. Select a drug that may be prescribed for a patient being discharged following hospitalization (identify the patient's condition). State the potential problems that might occur in reaction to the drug and the action you would take in response.

The nurse in psychiatric services will be involved in a variety of therapeutic methods in the treatment of emotional illness. The extent of participation in treatment depends on the philosophy of the psychiatric facility and the effectiveness of the nurse's relationship with the patient.

INDIVIDUAL PSYCHOTHERAPY

Individual psychotherapy is a process that uses a relationship between therapist and patient to identify, examine, and achieve understanding of the patient's problem. Its purpose is to provide support necessary to establish insight into thoughts, feelings, and behavior. Through this process the patient is better able to establish and maintain interpersonal relationships and deal more effectively with anxiety. Despite recent attacks on psychotherapy as an effective treatment method, the therapeutic process serves to reinforce the patient's confidence in the therapist. The role of the psychotherapist requires specialization in the field of the psychodynamics of human development and behavior and in the science of psychotherapy.

GROUP PSYCHOTHERAPY

Traditionally, group therapy is used to describe a method in which several individuals attend a specified number of meetings directed by a therapist or co-therapist. The purpose of group therapy is to provide group members with insight into and awareness of thoughts, feelings, and behaviors. The advantages to this form of therapy are derived from the fact that emotional problems involve feelings and behavior that are directed toward others. Through feedback and support from the group, individuals are encouraged to change behavior and formulate new, effective interpersonal relationships with others.

The types of groups presently utilized include problem-solving groups, remotivation groups, re-education groups, personality reconstruction groups, and support groups.

FAMILY THERAPY

The primary aim of family therapy is to treat the family as a social system. Family therapy is a form of group therapy in which the patient and members of the family work together to achieve insight into their emotional conflicts. The roots of emotional problems are regularly found in the complex interpersonal interactions that take place within the home. Conflicts between family members often lead to communication breakdown, making it difficult, if not impossible, for family members to work out their problems without assistance. The goals of family therapy are to assist family members to identify each other's needs, to reduce or resolve family conflicts and anxieties, to develop appropriate role relationships, to assist individual members to cope effectively with conflicts within the family unit, and to promote an emotional climate conducive to the health and growth of the family.

MILIEU THERAPY

Milieu therapy is defined as "a scientific manipulation of the environment aimed at producing changes in the personality of the patient." This form of therapy is designed to use the total environment, including physical surroundings, staff members, and a specific program plan that aims at achieving, supporting, and maintaining the mental health of the patient. The program plan includes the living environment and experiences in the community with the expectation that patients will work with staff toward a goal of independence, competence in self-care, and satisfaction in daily living. Staff members follow a carefully designed and consistent plan to encourage independence and initiative, assisting patients where necessary but providing opportunities that require the patient to make choices.

SOMATIC THERAPY

Somatic therapy is the treatment of the emotionally ill person by physiologic means. Electroconvulsive therapy, insulin coma therapy, psychosurgery, orthomolecular treatment, and hydrotherapy are other forms of treatment that may supplement medications and psychotherapy. Somatic treatments are generally characterized by their effect on the patterns of patient behavior in ways that make patients who are extremely anxious or depressed more accessible to psychotherapy or other therapeutic plans.

Specific nursing procedures in somatic treatments are dictated by the policies and procedures of the treatment facility. However, nursing management requires a high degree of observational skill and knowledge of emergency measures. Personnel should know the prescribed measures and the location of emergency equipment and supplies. Any unusual symptoms or reactions should be reported at once.

Patients receiving electronic therapy usually show confusion, disorientation, and loss of memory following treatment. The support given by the nursing staff during periods of confusion, and the help that assists the patient with reorientation promote more healthy patterns of behavior.

THE THERAPEUTIC COMMUNITY*

As a treatment method, the therapeutic community model is used to deal with a variety of emotional behavior problems. The program is useful in the treatment of substance abusers, as well as short- and long-term institutionalized patients. (The young as well as the elderly benefit from the caring environment.)

The primary goal of the therapeutic community is to assist the individual to develop a sense of responsibility toward self and others. This is accomplished in a homelike atmosphere where patients and staff share the responsibilities of daily living. Each person has the opportunity to explore feelings and behaviors and to examine the effect of the behavior on others in the community. Opportunities are provided to try out new behaviors in a safe environment. The use of the principles of behavior modification by members of the group in decision making assists all patients to become more responsible, independent, and self-directed. Caring and sharing become guiding principles for all participants.

The nurse as a member of the community serves as a role model and consultant to patients. The ability of the staff to be open and caring and to share thoughts and feelings helps set the tone for this humanistic program.

PSYCHOTHERAPEUTIC DRUGS

The use of tranquilizing drugs is an invaluable addition to milieu factors on which contemporary psychiatric care is based. Drugs alone should not be thought of as a cure for emotional illness but as agents to alleviate certain symptoms and allow individuals to participate in other forms of treatment.

NURSING CONSIDERATIONS

Communication with patients for whom the psychopharmacologic agents are prescribed is essential. Patients need to feel confident that nurses understand their concerns, especially when unusual discomforts are associated with the medication. Keen observation of symptoms that reveal side effects about which patients should be informed must be reported for patients' comfort and safety. A "not to worry" comment is inappropriate and may

---

*This section was written by Anne Peet, B.S., R.N., Supervisor, The Therapeutic Community, Hancock Geriatric Treatment Center, Williamsburg, Virginia.

increase the level of anxiety or distress already being experienced, even when the discomfort is obviously minor. It is essential for the patient to avoid activities that are hazardous to safety. Most patients can understand and accept warnings about the use of alcohol, driving a car, and climbing ladders. Dizziness, nausea, and many of the other possible side effects that cause discomfort will usually be reported by the patient, and should be reported to the supervisor or physician. Confusion and tremors may not be reported or may frighten the patient, who tries to ignore or hide the symptoms. On the hospital unit, many of the side effects can be observed by nurses even before the patient complains of them. If a patient is being treated in a clinic, a day-care facility, or is on medication at home, it will be useful to give both the patient and a family member a written sheet with a list of possible side effects and instructions concerning action to be taken if side effects occur. This involves the patient in responsibility for personal health practices, *and* may reduce the patient's anxiety associated with lack of knowledge of what is happening.

Example: Thorazine was prescribed for a man with a chronic schizophrenic disorder who was living at home with a companion. The patient was warned about excessive exposure to the sun, but neither he nor his companion remembered this, since neither of them thought they were exposed to much sun in their daily activities. The man developed a severe rash on his hands, and immediately thought he had acquired pellagra. He was in an increased state of anxiety until he saw his physician.

Classifications of Psychotherapeutic Agents

Two classes of psychotherapeutic agents are discussed in this chapter: *tranquilizers* and *mood modifiers*. Tranquilizers formerly were classified as being of major or minor origin. Currently it is generally agreed that the major tranquilizers are the *neuroleptics* or ataractic agents. Neuroleptic agents are used in the treatment of psychotic symptoms. Minor tranquilizers are classified as *anxiolytics* or antineurotic agents. These drugs are used to relieve mild to moderate anxiety and symptoms accompanying neurotic states. The anxiolytic or antineurotic drugs are not considered effective in the treatment of psychotic symptoms. *Mood modifiers* or psychostimulants are agents used in the treatment of depression. Psychostimulants are made up of the antidepressant and antimanic agents. Their effect is to stimulate energy-producing actions that elevate the mood of depressed individuals, or control manic episodes in manic-depressive illness.

TRANQUILIZERS

Neuroleptics or Antipsychotic Agents (Major Tranquilizers)

The use of antipsychotic agents has brought about major changes in the treatment of emotional illness. Rauwolfia alkaloids were the first pharmacologic substances used as neuroleptic agents. Preparations of this substance are thought to have been used in India for centuries for the treatment of various illnesses. At present, rauwolfia alkaloids are seldom used except for their antihypertensive properties.

The neuroleptic drugs are divided into several chemically distinct groups. These compounds are characterized by their calming effect on disturbed behavior and improvement of the mood of psychotic individuals, without causing dependence or marked sedation. Chemically the neuroleptics are significantly more potent and toxic than the antianxiety agents. Depression of the lower brain centers, depressed general motor activity, and extrapyramidal symptoms are characteristic of their effects on the central nervous system.

The most widely used antipsychotic drugs are the *phenothiazines*. It is believed that the most potent of these have the highest incidence of extrapyramidal side effects. Others are known to possess the greatest incidence of sedation and hypotension. An additional characteristic of the phenothiazine group is its antiemetic properties. Generally, the antiemetic potency is equivalent to the antipsychotic properties.

Neuroleptic agents (Major tranquilizers)
Phenothiazines
Thorazine (chlorpromazine hydrochloride)
Vesprin (triflupromazine hydrochloride)
Mellaril (thioridazine hydrochloride)
Serentil (mesoridazine besylate)
Quide (piperacetazine)
Stelazine (trifluoperazine hydrochloride)
Tindal (acetophenazine maleate)
Repoise (butaperazine maleate)
Prolixin (fluphenazine hydrochloride)
Trilafon (perphenazine)
Compazine (prochlorperazine maleate)
Taractan (chlorprothixene)
Navane (thiothixene hydrochloride)

Haldol (haloperidol)
Loxitane (loxapine succinate)

Nursing Considerations

Remain with the patient until medication has been swallowed.

Instruct the patient to sit or lie down when dizzy or faint. Advise getting up slowly from a lying-down position and sitting on the side of the bed for a minute or two before starting to walk. If in distress, call a nurse.

Observe patient for slurred speech, dizziness, and ataxia. These symptoms indicate acute intoxication and should be reported to supervisor or to presiding physician at once.

Advise the patient not to drive or operate dangerous equipment or machinery without approval of the physician. Also caution patient not to climb ladders.

Instruct the patient to avoid exposure to excessive sunlight, to wear a hat and long sleeves in the sun.

Inform patients of possible allergic reactions and side effects that are frequently associated with tranquilizers. Identify these to patient.

Advise the patient to avoid drinking any alcoholic beverage, even lite beer.

Advise patient to consult medical supervisor if persistent insomnia or confusion occurs.

Monitor patient's intake and output and observe for signs of abdominal distention, constipation, and urinary retention.

Instruct that neuroleptic agents sometimes interfere with sexual performance in men and can be relieved by medication adjustment.

Observe and report any menstrual irregularities, lactation, increased libido, or breast engorgement in women.

Instruct patients to have regular eye examinations. Observe for any signs of visual difficulties and report this to supervisor or physician.

Advise patients that abrupt cessation of neuroleptic agents may result in nausea, vomiting, headaches, sweating tachycardia, and insomnia.

Anxiolytics or Antineurotic Agents (Minor Tranquilizers)

The anxiolytic drugs are a new classification for the antianxiety agents or minor tranquilizers. These tranquilizers are used in the treatment of mild to moderate anxiety. They are also prescribed for conditions requiring muscle relaxation and for stress associated with environmental factors. Higher doses are sometimes prescribed for the treatment of acute agitation in psychotic individuals. These agents are also frequently utilized as an additional therapy in the treatment of rheumatoid arthritis, selected convulsive disorders, alcohol withdrawal, premenstrual tension, angina pectoris, and asthma, and to induce sleep as premedication for cardioversion and surgery.

All anxiolytic agents can cause physical and psychologic dependency. Abrupt withdrawal of high doses may result in convulsions, coma or, even death. If an individual has received large doses of these medications, the physician usually orders gradually reduced doses over a period of weeks or months.

The side effects usually associated with these drugs include drowsiness, allergic reactions, blood dyscrasias, itching, lowered tolerance to alcohol, nausea, vomiting, constipation, generalized weakness, slurred speech, confusion, urinary frequency, bronchial spasms, headaches, hypotension, dizziness, and anaphylactic reactions. These drugs are almost always contraindicated in children under the age of five and for persons known to be hypersensitive.

Anxiolytic agents (Minor tranquilizers)
  Benzodiazepines
    Librium (chlordiazepoxide hydrochloride)
    Tranxene (chlorazepate dipotassium)
    Azene (chlorazepate monopotassium)
    Valium (diazepam)
    Ativan (lorazepam)
    Serax (oxazepam)
    Restoril (temazepam)
    Centrax (prazepam)
  Nonbenzodiazepines
    Tybatran (tybamate)
    Equanil (meprobamate)
    Sinequan (doxepin hydrochloride)
    Vistaril, Atarax (hydroxyzine hydrochloride)

MOOD MODIFIERS

The mood modifiers are made up of three chemically distinct groups of agents. They include the *monoamine oxidase inhibitors, tricyclic antidepressants,* and *lithium salts.*

Monoamine Oxidase Inhibitors

Monoamine oxidase (MAO) inhibitors were first synthesized in the early 1950s. They were also the first antidepressants introduced for the treatment of depression. The exact mechanism of action of the MAO inhibitors is not understood. They are used primarily in the treatment of personality disorders and psychoses characterized by marked depression, in involutional melancholia, and in depressive reactions in manic-depressive psychoses.

The prescription of MAO inhibitors is contraindicated with known hypersensitivity, altered liver function, history of renal disease, hyperthyroidism, epilepsy, arteriosclerosis, cerebrovascular disease, paranoid schizophrenia, glaucoma, hypernatremia, cardiovascular disease, and atonic colitis.

Monoamine oxidase inhibitors
Nardil (phenelzine sulfate)
Marplan (isocarboxazid)
Parnate (tranylcypromine sulfate)

Nursing Considerations
Advise patient not to take any other medication without medical supervision during, or two to three weeks after, therapy.

MAO inhibitors should never be administered with tricyclic antidepressants, such as Tofranil, Elavil, and Norpramin.

Instruct patient that foods rich in tyramine should be avoided. Provide patient with information relative to foods rich in tyramine, such as cheese, wine, or anything aged.

Observe patient's vital signs frequently and note hypertension, which may indicate discontinuance of therapy.

Advise patient to avoid drinking beverages containing stimulants. Coffee, Coca-Cola, and alcoholic drinks should be omitted during treatment.

Observe patient for peripheral edema or other symptoms indicative of congestive heart failure.

Observe patient's red-green vision for early signs of optic damage.

Monitor patient's intake and output for possible urinary retention.

Tricyclic Antidepressants

The tricyclic group of antidepressants do not inhibit the enzyme monoamine oxidase; for that reason they are frequently referred to as non-MAO antidepressants. Chemically, the tricyclic antidepressants are similar to the phenothiazines. Their actions include anticholinergic, antihistaminic, anti-serotonin, anticonvulsant, hypotensive, and sedative effects. Tricyclic anti-depressants are chiefly used in the treatment of endogenous and reactive depression. Generally, they are preferred over MAO inhibitors because it is felt that they are less toxic. They are used occasionally in the treatment of enuresis in children. They may also be used when electroconvulsive ther-apy is indicated. Side effects frequently encountered with tricyclic antide-pressants include atropine-like reactions (such as dry mouth, headaches, muscle tremors, ataxia, insomnia, heartburn, tachycardia, nausea, vomit-ing, orthostatic hypotension), allergic reactions, acute mania, parkinsonism-like symptoms, agitation, and anxiety.

Tricyclic antidepressants
Tofranil (imipramine hydrochloride)
Elavil (amitriptyline hydrochloride)
Norpramin (desipramine hydrochloride)
Aventyl (nortriptyline hydrochloride)
Vivactil (protriptyline hydrochloride)
Surmontil (trimipramine maleate)

Nursing Considerations
Advise patient not to take any medication without medical supervision dur-ing, or two to three weeks after, therapy.
Advise patient that sudden discontinuance of therapy may result in symp-toms characteristic of withdrawal. Identify these symptoms, giving patient a list, if appropriate.

Lithium Salts

Lithium carbonate for the purpose of this chapter will be considered a mood modifier. Generally, it has been classified as a miscellaneous or anti-psychotic agent. I consider it a mood modifier because of its effect on the mood of manic individuals. This agent has been exclusively used in the treatment of the manic phase of manic-depressive psychoses. The mode of action is unknown. Serum lithium levels require frequent monitoring be-cause the difference between therapeutic and toxic dose levels is narrow. Early signs of lithium intoxication include the following: vomiting, diarrhea, drowsiness, and ataxia. (To reduce the possibility of lithium intoxication, sodium levels must also be monitored and maintained within normal limits.) Other side effects that may be associated with lithium therapy include thirst, polyuria, fine tremors, anorexia, slurred speech, fatigue, and malaise. Severe reactions can be characterized by convulsions, oliguria, circulation failure, coma, and death.

Antimanic agents
Lithium carbonate

Nursing Considerations
The patient should be warned that if diarrhea, nausea, vomiting, drowsiness, and muscular weakness occur, the medical supervisor should be contacted, and lithium therapy should be discontinued.

Advise patient that serum lithium level must be frequently monitored because the difference between therapeutic and toxic levels is narrow.

Advise the patient to avoid consumption of excessive amounts of salt.

Advise the patient that excessive sweating or diarrhea may indicate the need for medical consultation.

Instruct the patient to maintain fluid intake of 2 to 3 liters per day.

Advise the patient to avoid excessive physical activities.

LEARNING ACTIVITIES

1. Request information about the number and types of psychotherapeutic groups being conducted on the unit or service to which you are assigned. Study the purposes and goals of each of the therapies. If possible, secure information concerning how patients are selected. Identify professional personnel serving as therapist and co-therapist, or team leader and members. It is likely that a number of nursing personnel assigned to the unit will not be directly involved in the therapeutic group. How is pertinent information concerning their relationships with the patients being transmitted to them?
2. Arrange to talk with a patient who is a member of a therapeutic community group. Report comments and reactions. Focus your role on listening and observing. Report your discussion to class members.
3. You are assigned to work with a patient for whom a psychotherapeutic drug is prescribed. Observe the patient for evidence of signs or symptoms of behavior suggested in the description of the drug, and its possible effects. Record your observations as well as any concerns or questions of the patient about the effects being experienced. Describe your response, and any action you took. Prepare a summary of your observa-

tions and discussion with the patient for class discussion. Include the symptom list you gave the patient for class review and evaluation.

4. Assume that a relative or friend has been hospitalized for treatment and is being discharged with instructions to continue a neuroleptic drug. You are expected to counsel the patient concerning the medication. List the signs and symptoms you would be concerned with, and describe the action you would take in the event certain symptoms (identify them) occur.

BIBLIOGRAPHY

ALBANESE, JA: *Nurses' Drug Reference.* McGraw-Hill, New York, 1979.

AMERICAN PSYCHIATRIC ASSOCIATION: *Diagnostic and Statistical Manual of Mental Disorders (DSM-III).* The Association, Washington, DC, 1980.

BERGERSEN, BS AND KRUG, EE: *Pharmacology in Nursing.* CV Mosby, St Louis, 1979.

CARTER, FM: *Psychosocial Nursing,* ed 3. Macmillan, New York, 1981.

Diazepam as a Muscle Relaxant. The Medical Letter 15:1, 1973.

GOTH, A: *Medical Pharmacology,* ed 19. CV Mosby, St Louis, 1981.

GOVONI, LE AND HAYES, JE: *Drugs and Nursing Implications.* Appleton-Century-Crofts, New York, 1979.

IRONS, PD: *Psychotropic Drugs and Nursing Intervention.* McGraw-Hill, New York, 1978.

MERENESS, D AND TAYLOR, CM: *Essentials of Psychiatric Nursing,* ed 10. CV Mosby, St Louis, 1978.

PEPLAU, HF: *Interpersonal Relations in Nursing.* GP Putnam's Sons, New York, 1952.

Physicians' Desk Reference, ed 37. Medical Economics, Oradell, NJ, 1983.

SCHOU, M: *Lithium in Psychiatric Therapy and Prophylaxis.* J Psychiatr Res 6:67, 1968.

Cassette tapes

Century Celebration Cassette Tapes, Eastern Audio Association, Inc., Oakland Center, 8980 Route 108, Columbia, MD, 21045.

82238-080 (G). *New Programs for Old People: Psychiatric Nursing as a Subspecialty.* Kaplan, S.

82238-090 (H). *Ethnic Minorities in Psychiatric Nursing: Patients and Personnel.* Murillo-Rohde, I.

82238-120 (L). *Individual Therapy: An Update on the 1974 State of the Art in Psychiatric Nursing Conference.* Lego, S.

82238-130 (M). *Milieu Therapy: An Update on the 1974 State of the Art in Psychiatric Nursing Conference.* Sills, G.

82238-140 (N). *Family Therapy: An Update on the State of the Art in Psychiatric Nursing Conference.* Smoyak, S.

82238-150 (O). *Group Therapy: An Update on the State of the Art in Psychiatric Nursing Conference.* White, E.

82238-200 (S). *The Nurse and the Alcoholic: Redefining an Historically Ambivalent Relationship.* Naegle, M.

CHAPTER 7   *ANXIETY DISORDERS*

LEARNING OBJECTIVES

Study of this chapter should prepare the student to:
1. Define anxiety.
2. Identify the various forms of anxiety disorders.
3. Describe the symptoms and behaviors associated with each disorder.
4. State nursing interventions appropriate with persons experiencing anxiety that interferes with usual activities.

Anxiety is a common human experience that is often a motivating force in successful and rewarding productivity. A person reporting to a new position or facing an unfamiliar experience feels anxious. Even the most skilled and articulate politician feels anxious before an important public appearance. Control of anxious feelings by various adjustment techniques keeps a person functioning in normal daily activities. Anxiety that produces an extreme feeling of inner tension interferes with normal daily activities and may result in serious anxiety disorders.

CHARACTERISTICS OF ANXIETY DISORDERS

Anxiety disorders* are characterized by a disturbing anticipation of danger. This feeling may be focused on a specific object, activity, or event perceived as a threat to one's life, status, or security. The degree of anxiety may range from a feeling of unease to panic, creating a crisis for the individual. The sudden onset of a serious illness, a critical accident, or the death of a loved one may produce anxiety that causes sleeplessness and other symptoms to which the individual cannot readily adjust. An event that a person is convinced will alter the family structure, lifestyle, or standing in the community may produce a level of anxiety that makes a person feel completely helpless.

TYPES OF ANXIETY DISORDERS

Free-floating Anxiety

Free-floating anxiety is characterized by a vague sense of dread that something terrible is about to happen. An attack may occur as a sudden onset of *panic* accompanied by physical symptoms such as difficulty in breathing, trembling, chest pains, and nausea.

Phobias

A phobia is described as persistent irrational fear of a specific object, activity, or situation. A fear of insects or of riding a Ferris wheel may have no important effect on the daily life of a person since it is not necessary for the person to handle insects or ride in a Ferris wheel. If the fear involves an object or situation that interferes with the work role or essential activities of daily living, treatment becomes necessary.

Obsessive-Compulsive Form

The obsessive-compulsive form is characterized by ritualistic behavior, such as checking and rechecking the locking of doors, compulsive hand

---

*Categories of anxiety disorders are adapted from *Diagnostic and Statistical Manual of Mental Disorders (DSM-III)*, American Psychiatric Association, 1980.

washing, excessive use of toilet paper, and other repetitious acts. These activities are likely to interfere with work, with the maintenance of the home, and with social and interpersonal relationships. The onset occurs early in life and tends to persist.

Example: A 30-year-old woman with a responsible position could not get to her job on time because she was concerned that she had left the gas jet on her kitchen stove open. She expressed alarm that she might be responsible for "blowing up" the apartment house where she lived. Her return to check often occurred as many as 16 or 17 times before she could leave the building. She repeatedly cautioned other workers in the building where she worked to "be careful, don't get hurt on the way home." She was able to get some relief by extended psychotherapy.

Hypochondriacal Form

The hypochondriacal form is characterized by a persistent fear of disease. The person is constantly preoccupied with the discovery of new symptoms and the dire effect this will have on future health and welfare. The preoccupation with symptoms and ailments may seriously interfere with interpersonal, social, and work relationships.

Example: A young man purchased many over-the-counter medicines to relieve symptoms suggested by television advertisements. He frequently spoke of his fear that he might transmit "something" to others, and therefore took the medicine as a precaution.

NURSING CONSIDERATIONS

Persons who experience anxiety disorders may require emergency treatment only in the event of a panic attack caused by a situation that cannot be successfully resolved. If a state of chronic immobilizing anxiety has developed over an extended period and has become increasingly severe in spite of the efforts of a physician and the family, hospitalization or mental health center admission may be required. Many of the persons who are victims of anxiety disorders have been frequent seekers of health services because of continuous concern with physical health.

If hospitalization is required, the treatment program may be brief and intensive, but the patient who has suffered this level of anxiety will probably wish to continue a therapeutic relationship that provides continuing support. When discharge from the hospital is planned, the evaluations by the patient and staff members will determine whether referral to a psychiatric nurse, a physician, a mental health center or clinic, or a community nursing service is indicated. The person to whom the patient is being referred or a staff member from the agency may attend the discharge conference to get acquainted with the patient and acquire information to ensure continuity of appropriate service. The patient whose anxiety has been out of control to the extent that hospitalization was required may continue to be a potential suicide risk, and needs a ready source of help to cope with crises until comfortable about his or her ability to do so. These are the patients who are sometimes considered problem patients who should be able to "shape up." If a truly trusting therapeutic relationship can be established with a health worker who is available but firm and patient, the person may be able to cope with the disorder in a more comfortable manner.

Patient's Symptoms and Behavior	*Suggested Nursing Interventions*
Appears threatened by "unknown danger."	Encourage patient to share feelings of anxiety and concern. Reassurance is important. Continuing presence of or immediate access to nursing personnel is best means of reassurance.
Demands for attention may be excessive.	Be alert to what the patient is trying to communicate; may be fearful of being left alone.
May dominate conversation by preoccupation with physical symptoms.	Be supportive, but avoid reinforcing physical complaints, such as frequent taking of pulse. This only serves to increase preoccupation with symptoms.
Excessive concern about or neglect of personal hygiene and physical appearance may be associated with ritualistic behavior.	Give patient appropriate assistance and support. Emphasize any changes because these may be important indications of patient's progress.
Treatment may include psychotherapeutic drugs and/or psychotherapy and milieu therapy, as indicated.	Be prompt with all prescribed treatment and medications. Refer to Chapter 6 to learn indications for report of the effects of medication.
Schedule daily activities planned in accord with patient's treatment program.	Encourage patient to participate in planning program of activities. Seek opportunities to communicate your expectation of patient's recovery. Remove patient from any situation in which anxiety becomes intolerable.

LEARNING ACTIVITIES

1. Make a list of events and activities that create anxiety for you on the left of a sheet of paper. List the ways you deal with your anxiety on the right.

Study this profile and think of ways you might change your behavior if you believe change would make you more comfortable. You may not wish to discuss this with anyone else. Feel free to choose what you will do with it.

2. Request assignment to a patient who is experiencing anxiety that interferes with activities and requires treatment. Plan nursing care with the patient and solicit the patient's comments and suggestions. Use the nursing process.

3. List the chief goals of the nursing care plan and explain your reasons to the patient. Use the questions below as a guide.

Is there a special time or an event that seems to increase anxiety?

Are specific situations and events that provoke increased anxiety understood by the patient?

Are you able to discuss these situations or events with the patient?

What special activities are planned for channeling the patient's anxiety and promoting interest in other people or things?

What particular feeling did this patient's behavior evoke within you? How did you handle these feelings?

Summarize the steps and rationale for your nursing plan. Present the plan to your instructor and classmates for evaluation.

BIBLIOGRAPHY

Anxiety, Recognition and Intervention (programmed instruction). Am J Nurs 65:127, 1965.

BAILEY, DS AND DREYER, SO: *Therapeutic Approaches to the Care of the Mentally Ill.* FA Davis, Philadelphia, 1977.

CARTER, FM: *Psychosocial Nursing,* ed 3. Macmillan, New York, 1981.

CIUCA, R, DOWNIE, CS, AND MORRIS, M: *When a disaster happens, how do you meet emotional needs?* Am J Nurs 77:454–456, March, 1977.

LIPKIN, GB AND COHEN, RG: *Effective Approaches to Patients' Behavior,* ed 2. Springer, New York, 1980.

CHAPTER 8   *AFFECTIVE DISORDERS*

LEARNING OBJECTIVES

Study of this chapter should prepare the student to:
1. Identify the predominant characteristics of the affective disorders.
2. State the symptoms and behaviors of individuals in the
   A. Manic phase
   B. Depressive phase
3. List the nursing interventions you would use in your work with patients in the
   A. Manic phase
   B. Depressive phase
4. Describe the current treatments used, and indicate the reactions to treatments which should be observed and reported.

The affective disorders* range from mild to severe episodes of mania and/or depression.

---

*Categories taken from *Diagnostic and Statistical Manual of Mental Disorders (DSM-III)*, American Psychiatric Association, 1980.

CHARACTERISTICS OF AFFECTIVE DISORDERS

Major affective disorders are characterized by disturbances of mood accompanied by mania or depression which is not due to other mental or physical disorders. These conditions are among the oldest recognized mental disorders. Early Greek and Roman physicians prescribed soothing baths, exercise, and soft music in a quiet setting to calm the distraught. Saul's depression and his plea for release from "evil spirits" is described in the Bible, First Samuel, chapter 16. The young David was dispatched, at Saul's request, to play his harp as a means of calming and comforting him. In the 20th century, Clifford Beers wrote of his 3-year battle with manic depressive disorder in his book *A Mind That Found Itself.* He also founded the National Committee for Mental Hygiene, an example of the industry and leadership often associated with the manic personality.

Until the advent of electroconvulsive treatment during the 1930s and the use of psychotherapeutic drugs some years later, hydrotherapy, exercise, occupational therapy, and music continued to be used in treatment programs.

The onset of these disorders usually occurs during the years between 18 and 29. Episodes may recur at varying intervals into the middle or later years. Elderly patients may suffer attacks of *involutional melancholia*, a disorder characterized by agitated depression and a high risk of suicide.

MANIC PHASE

During the early stages, the individual may display an expansive wit, require little sleep, wear clothing that is more colorful than usual, monopolize conversation, and advance imaginative but unrealistic plans for accumulating wealth, prestige, or power. If the change of mood and behavior is recognized as a signal for further disability and the individual is willing to accept treatment, hospitalization may not be necessary.

During the *acute manic phase,* the individual is extremely hyperactive and distractible. The flow of ideas is continuous and rapid with little recognizable sequence of content. Weight loss is common because the patient is too busy to eat, and dehydration may be severe. The irritability that occurs when someone tries to interrupt is disturbing to other patients when space is shared, such as in dayrooms or TV lounges. These patients often produce volumes of written material. The content may include schemes and contracts sent to government or industrial leaders, or letters containing inappropriate proposals or embarrassing propositions to family and friends. Projects may be undertaken that cause inconvenience or embarrassment to others.

Example: A 47-year-old man being treated in a suburban hospital passed a dairy farm while out for a walk. It suddenly occurred to him that the hospital could save money and serve really fresh milk if it owned dairy cows and allowed the patients to do the milking. He convinced the dairy farmer that he was an agent of the hospital and had come to purchase part of the herd. His offer was so attractive that the farmer could not refuse, and agreed to deliver the cows to the hospital where a check would be waiting the delivery. Both the hospital and the farmer were surprised when the cows were delivered the next morning. Following this event, the patient was accompanied by a staff member on his morning walk.

Before current forms of treatment were available, patients were frequently hospitalized for several months during an episode. A treatment regimen that included attention to nutritional needs, planned exercise, and hydrotherapy was used to re-establish a healthy physical condition. Psychotherapy was aimed at assisting the patient to gain insight and modify his or her lifestyle to cope with recurrences.

Example: A remarkably competent woman in her late thirties had appeared for treatment in a psychiatric hospital about every 2 or 3 years since the age of 27. Her episodes of mania usually lasted about 4 months. On admission, she was loud and boisterous, and extremely distractible. She suffered a substantial weight loss, and was dehydrated. She slept little and paced about much of the night. Her disturbed behavior appeared to terminate almost as suddenly as it began. On Wednesday afternoon, a staff nurse served her a snack consisting of a sandwich and a glass of milk. As she appeared to reach for the tray, she picked up the glass of milk and poured it over the head of the staff nurse. On Friday of that same week, the same staff nurse was making rounds with the psychiatrist. When the psychiatrist entered the patient's room she said, "I think I'll be ready to return to work next week." The reply, "If you feel you are ready, I will write discharge orders." The next week she was back at her job.

DEPRESSED PHASE

The onset of the depressed phase may occur gradually. The person works longer hours but accomplishes little. He or she becomes increasingly tense and anxious. This may occur following a significant loss or a threatening or disruptive illness.

In the *profoundly depressed phase,* the predominant mood is loss of interest or pleasure in all activity. The person is sad, cries easily, and feels discouraged, depressed, and hopeless. Loss or increase in appetite results in substantial weight change. Sleep is disturbed. The individual has difficulty getting to sleep and may claim lack of sleep. Even with sleep the person awakens feeling tired and listless. Psychomotor agitation, pacing, hand wringing, and picking at cuticles and skin are common. Expressing hopelessness about the likelihood of being forgiven for "past sins" are common. Agitation and discomfort increase if an effort is made by family members, friends, or health personnel to deny the reality of any guilt or to belittle the hopelessness.

Example: A hospitalized patient who was profoundly depressed appeared at the nursing supervisor's office one morning saying, "Please don't assign Miss _____ to work with me. She bounces into my room, all smiles and good cheer when I am so depressed I can hardly get out of bed, dress myself, and get through the day. I know she means well, but I cannot tolerate her cheerfulness when I am so depressed.

The depressed person may consider suicide as the only way out. During the period of profound depression the person may be unable to plan and carry out a suicide. The greater danger comes when the depression is lifting, but the person continues to have periods of depression and hopelessness.

The person whose depression follows a significant loss usually continues to experience periods of overwhelming grief and deprivation until the grieving process has been accomplished. As the early close and frequent attention of friends and family lessens, the risk of suicide is increased. Only when the person takes up earlier interests and activities can the potential for suicide be discounted.

Example: A husband whose wife had died of cancer following 30 years of a happy marriage visited her grave almost daily for some weeks. After several months passed his visits to the cemetery became less frequent. His children also spent less time with him. During a visit following a period when he had not visited for 2 or 3 weeks, he went to the gravesite, knelt, and shot himself.

Current treatments have lessened the burden of prolonged depressive episodes. Early treatment and education that assists persons prone to depression or manic depressive disorders when events overwhelm them, has significantly decreased the loss of productive capacity for such persons.

Example: A severely depressed man was admitted to a psychiatric hospital following the loss of his construction business. He sat and stared, occasionally bemoaning his failure to provide adequately for his family. He responded only minimally when approached by staff members. The psychiatric director who had been tentatively planning some remodeling of a building on the hospital grounds casually approached the patient as he sat staring into space, and mentioned the plans. The patient did not respond. In a few days the director passed the porch as the patient sat looking profoundly depressed. Ostensibly enroute to look at the building plans for remodeling, the director stopped to chat, and told the patient he was looking further into the remodeling potential and, as an afterthought upon leaving, said, "I could certainly use an expert to help me plan." The director noted a slight expression of interest by the patient and went away. In a few days the director passed that way again. The patient mentioned the remodeling. When the patient was invited to accompany the director, he did and, after some reluctance, let the psychiatrist know that he would think about tackling the job. As the work progressed, the patient, feeling worthy and competent again, returned to a management position with a construction firm near his home.

NURSING CONSIDERATIONS

Patients in both the manic and depressed phase require consistent responses from nursing personnel. These patients are rarely, if ever, confused or disoriented.

The patient in the manic phase tests the calm resolve of staff members by unexpected acts of provocation, by playful manipulation, and by persuasion.

The depressed suicidal patient may request privacy and quiet, complaining of sleepiness after being awake all night. This may secure the time to commit suicide with a full bottle of sedatives an uninformed relative or friend brought as an act of helpfulness when the patient complained of difficulty in getting to sleep.

The Manic Patient	*Suggested Nursing Interventions*
Hyperactive and distractible. May ask staff for special favors.	Plan brief periods of activity that do not require continued concentration.
Loud and boisterous language in presence of other patients.	Be consistent and honest at all times.
Non-stop talking; irritability when interrupted.	Plan activities that remove patient from group, and reduce exposure to stimuli.
Restlessness.	Include physical exercise to use excess energy. Use kind, firm manner when approaching patient.
Check weight for loss. May be "too busy" to eat.	Select highly nutritious foods that patients like. Provide snacks between meals.

Check patient's attention to hygiene.

May engage other patients and staff in "get rich quick" or other manipulative schemes.
May appear in outlandish clothing to attract attention.

Be sure patient does not forget to brush teeth, bathe, and take time for bowel movements.
Listen, and report any evidence of activity to superior. Observe changes in mood and behavior, and report.
Assist patient with dress and make-up to minimize bizarre effects.

The Depressed Patient

Suggested Nursing Interventions

Responds slowly, attention limited.
Difficulty in decision making.

Tires easily.
May be agitated, pacing, and picking at skin and hair.
May avoid others, expressing unworthiness to associate.
May plan or consider suicide as depression lifts at intervals.

Allow time for response.
Present plans and information simply and clearly.
Allow time for rest.
Plan activities using hands. Remaining with patient may reduce agitation.
Arrange brief, casual contacts that do not require initial overt approach.
Be alert for clues and actions that vary from past behavior. If depression is lifting, observe closely for recurrence which discourages patient and provokes suicide attempt. Check any environmental hazards, remove objects, and check clothing that might be used in suicide attempt.

May not wish to see visitors, expressing feelings of not being worthy of attention or belief they are only curious about appearance.
May offer to do a menial task to pay for trouble he/she caused staff.

Remain with, or plan continuing observation to reassure patient, but do not try to "cheer up."

Allow to help, if possible, but with something that can be cited as real achievement that patient can accept.

Patients who experience affective disorders are usually productive persons, many holding responsible positions of leadership. With a combination of psychotherapeutic drugs and psychotherapy, these patients generally acquire insight into their mental health problem and continue with health supervision following discharge from hospitalization. They may receive continuing health care from a psychiatrist or psychiatric nurse in private practice, in a mental health center, or a clinic. If the patient has received treatment in a service facility or on a day-care or a regular basis, the treatment may continue. The goal of the patient and health service will be to continue to assist the patient to cope with stress and loss, in an increasingly healthy manner.

LEARNING ACTIVITIES

1. Request assignment to provide nursing care to:
   A. a patient in the manic phase
   B. a person who is profoundly depressed
   Use the nursing process to plan and carry out your plan of care. Involve the patient in planning, to the extent possible. Patient involvement is an important goal. Discuss your plan and report progress to your instructor. Use your plan and report for class discussion if possible.
2. If the patient is receiving medication, refer to the section Psychotherapeutic Drugs in Chapter 6 to learn what side effects you should watch for and record or report. If the patient is receiving psychotherapy, do not enter into discussions with the patient concerning the treatment unless specifically instructed. Report any questions or comments made to you by the patient.

BIBLIOGRAPHY

AMERICAN PSYCHIATRIC ASSOCIATION: *Diagnostic and Statistical Manual of Mental Disorders (DSM-III).* The Association, Washington, DC, 1980.

BAILEY, DS AND DREYER, SO: *Therapeutic Approaches to the Care of the Mentally Ill.* FA Davis, Philadelphia, 1977.

CARTER, FM: *Psychosocial Nursing,* ed 3. Macmillan, New York, 1981.

Depressive Disorders: Causes and Treatment. National Institute of Mental Health, US Department of Health and Human Services, Washington, DC, 1981.

PEPLAU, HF: *Interpersonal Relations in Nursing.* GP Putnam's Sons, New York, 1952.

Psychiatric Nursing Standards. Eastern State Hospital, Williamsburg, Va, 1982.

REGAN, P: *Brief psychotherapy of depression.* Am J Psychiatry 122:28, 1965.

SAXTON, DF AND HARING, PW: *Care of Patients with Emotional Problems,* ed 3. CV Mosby, St Louis, 1979.

WHITE, CL: *Nurse counseling with a depressed patient.* Am J Nurs 78:436–439, March, 1978.

CHAPTER 9   SCHIZOPHRENIC DISORDERS

LEARNING OBJECTIVES

Study of this chapter should prepare the student to:

1. State the reasons why schizophrenic disorders present a major health problem in the United States.

2. Define the behaviors characteristic of the onset of a schizophrenic disorder.

3. List the types of schizophrenic disorders described in the *Diagnostic and Statistical Manual of Mental Disorders (DSM-III)* of the American Psychiatric Association, and identify the disabling symptoms.

4. List the treatments in current use with schizophrenic patients.

5. Identify symptoms and behaviors and state the nursing interventions appropriate to assist patients in coping with these disorders.

6. List and describe some of the resources available in the community to provide continuing assistance to these persons.

Individuals who suffer schizophrenic disorders* constitute a major health problem in the United States. At least two million people are estimated to

---

*Categories taken from *Diagnostic and Statistical Manual of Mental Disorders (DSM-III)*, American Psychiatric Association, 1980.

require treatment annually. The onset generally occurs in adolescence or early adulthood and the disabling effects tend to persist over prolonged periods. The result may be chronic impairment or profound disability requiring repeated institutional or other protective supervision and care.

The specific causes of this group of disorders have not been confirmed by extensive investigation, but several theories are the subject of continuing research. The theories include the: (1) psychologic or experiential, (2) biologic, (3) organic, (4) vitamin deficiency, and (5) environmental or sociocultural.

CHARACTERISTICS OF SCHIZOPHRENIC DISORDERS

Patients who suffer from the schizophrenic disorders present a pattern of diminished or profound loss of contact with reality, a significant reduction in social and interpersonal relationships, and less or significantly lowered productive capacity.

The insidious onset characteristic of these disorders may be cause for concern by a variety of persons in frequent contact with the individual for an extended period before the serious nature of the disorder is recognized. The school nurse or a teacher may be the first to recognize that the gradual withdrawal of contact with reality, lessened interest in schoolwork, diminished social and interpersonal relationships, and the reduction or loss of productive capacity are distress signals. An inquiry about a cause for this behavior may elicit a flat, vague, or inappropriate response from the individual and denial or hostility from family members. Peer groups and coworkers may engage in mutual withdrawal or resort to ridicule or criticism because the individual appears to shirk responsibility in work or sports. Parents may be frustrated and angered by the behavior and seek to modify it by threats or coercion. When the person's withdrawn or frankly psychotic behavior becomes acute and disturbing to others in the home environment, school, or workplace, referral to a mental health center, a psychiatrist, or admission to a hospital usually occurs.

On admission to a hospital or clinic, these patients are frequently fearful, suspicious, and out of contact with reality. If a patient has been told by family members that they are going to a place other than a hospital, the patient may respond, on admission, with disturbed and disturbing behavior. If the onset is characterized by sudden explosive behavior associated with an overwhelming experience, the individual is probably agitated and may become combative.

TYPES OF SCHIZOPHRENIC DISORDERS

Five clinical types of schizophrenic disorders, each presenting serious symptoms, are described in the *Diagnostic and Statistical Manual of Mental Disorders (DSM-III)* of the American Psychiatric Association. This classification of the symptoms and behaviors is useful in effective planning for treatment and nursing intervention. However, it should be remembered that many patients present a mixture of symptoms.

Disorganized Type

The disorganized type presents the most severe personality disorganization, and has the most guarded prognosis for recovery. These patients are usually apathetic, with flat or inappropriate responses and silly or incoherent speech. They appear unable to relate fantasies to reality, and smile or laugh on receiving sad news. Their thoughts are usually dominated by fantasies. They may express or appear to respond to hallucinations (usually auditory) and delusions. The ability to plan or to carry out a task seems lost. They may make up words for which there seems to be no meaning. Their perception of body image may be distorted, and they may complain of physical symptoms. The characteristic regression exhibited by this type continues and confirms the chronicity.

Catatonic Type

The catatonic type is characterized by a sudden onset usually associated with a traumatic experience. The duration of the acute phase may be brief, but recurrent episodes are common. Posturing and stupor may be followed by sudden episodes of excitement and occasional destructive behavior. These patients are likely to become chronically impaired after several recurrent attacks.

Paranoid Type

The paranoid type may appear to occur as late as the thirties or early forties, but the suspicions and jealousies that characterize this disorder may have been present in a lesser degree much earlier. The person frequently continues to carry on a work schedule while gradually giving up all social and interpersonal relationships. These individuals are neat and well groomed, but may become careless if preoccupied by hallucinations and delusions of a persecutory nature. The establishment of a mutually trusting relationship is an essential element of treatment. The following is perhaps an uncommon, but true, example.

> *Example:* The patient and psychiatrist developed a mutual respect for each other during hospitalization which became a mutually trusting relationship. The patient had a responsible position in a distant city. When the patient and psychiatrist agreed on the return to work, they also made an agreement that if and when overwhelming anxiety and suspicions of co-workers occurred, the patient would telephone the psychiatrist. The hour-long telephone psychotherapy kept this patient on the job for many years, until retirement.

Residual Type

The residual type is described as "in partial remission." These individuals have a history of a previous episode but no longer exhibit obvious psychotic symptoms. They may be living at home or in residential facilities with minimum supervision. They usually show little initiative in activity, but create few problems in the environment. Some work at simple jobs, minimally self-supporting.

Undifferentiated Type

This category is used when a person exhibits a mixture of symptoms and cannot be classified in any one of the four types already described. *Acute undifferentiated* refers to a sudden onset of psychotic behavior, and *chronic undifferentiated* refers to longstanding withdrawn and eccentric behavior or mildly psychotic-like symptoms.

NURSING CONSIDERATIONS

Autism, suspiciousness, hallucinations, and delusions will usually cause persons experiencing a schizophrenic disorder to isolate themselves from others. On admission for treatment, the goal of the nurse is to establish a mutually trusting relationship with the patient. Even if the patient appears uninterested, make introductions to staff members and other patients in the environment. Give a schedule of meals and point out the location of the bathroom and the dining room. The patient does not usually respond to any gesture of closeness, especially to being touched. Simple statements should be designed to orient the patient, to assure acceptance, and to communicate recognition that stress and anxiety are appropriate feelings in the circumstances. It may be reassuring to say to the patient, "This is a hospital. I am a nurse. We will take care of you as long as you wish us to do so." Remember that this expressed commitment is an expectation of nurses held by many people and may be useful in an initial reality orientation in a confused and fearful patient.

The nurse should remember also that a patient who is frightened or near panic and confused by overwhelming events is often as sensitive to nonverbal communications as to what is being said. An expression of concerned interest in a person or an activity should be noted for follow-up. Clues to interest in any activity, such as piano playing or a game in progress on the unit, that might intercept withdrawn behavior should be reinforced. It is equally important for a patient, especially in the early phases of treatment, to be protected from stressful or threatening situations.

The nurse should not, at any time, turn away from the patient. Doing this may signal rejection and may cause the patient to commit an unpremeditated act of aggression that causes further disturbance and confusion.

The withdrawn patient will probably not initiate contacts with other patients or with staff members. The trusting relationships between the patient and staff members can be enhanced and the sense of isolation reduced by frequent casual recognition by staff members which communicates interest and concern.

Symptoms and behavior disturbances vary in severity and content for the clinical types described, but the characteristic loss of or diminished contact with reality and the reduction in social and interpersonal relationships and productive capacity are common to all types.

Nursing intervention has as an important goal the creation and management of an environment that promotes a re-establishment of contact with reality and social and interpersonal relationships, and a return to a productive capacity that assures a sense of satisfaction and accomplishment.

Psychotherapeutic drugs combined with psychotherapy, milieu therapy, or other treatments are usually prescribed. Nursing personnel must be aware of potential side effects of the drugs, and report promptly any evidence of drug interactions. Nursing personnel must also understand their responsibility for discussing the importance of follow-up instructions and contacting health personnel about their concerns when the patient is discharged with prescriptions.

Patient's Symptoms and Behavior	*Suggested Nursing Interventions*
Emotional responses shallow and inappropriate. May laugh on receiving	Be patient, recognize that behavior is in response to turmoil within. Use

disturbing message.

May become incoherent.

short simple statements about the present to draw attention to reality. Use concise nonauthoritative language to inform about activities and treatments prescribed. Be sure to address patients by name, using Mr., Mrs., or Miss—never first names or nicknames.

Disturbed thinking. Gestures and conversation may be in response to hallucinations and delusions, ignoring persons in the environment.
Impulsive and bizarre behavior should be anticipated as a possibility.

Be patient with the obvious problem in relating while preoccupied with inner thoughts, but remain with patient until attention is secured.
Be alert for restlessness which may be evidence that the patient is acutely distressed by inner thoughts. Allow the patient space; do not touch or get too near. If possible, distract the patient with something that you believe will attract the attention and reduce stress.

Has difficulty in relating to others when thinking is dominated by fantasies or when hallucinations are present.
Somatic complaints are common, but identity of symptoms vague.

Be alert for evidence that the patient is experiencing hallucinations. Inquire about what "voices" are saying, whether distressing or pleasant.
Ask about specific discomfort or symptoms. If unclear what the patient is telling you, request the information in a different way.

The Paranoid Patient

The patient experiencing the paranoid type of schizophrenic disorders presents some symptoms and behavior not usually associated with other types.

Patient's Symptoms and Behavior

Suggested Nursing Interventions

Usually views the environment as hostile and threatening. May accuse others without evidence: a spouse may be accused of infidelity or a friend of being out to "get me."

Observe to anticipate events or activities that appear upsetting, and modify plans to reduce possibility of aggressive or threatening acts. Do not argue, joke, or disagree, but be honest. Avoid laughing or whispering in patient's presence. Do whatever you tell patient you will do.

May refuse food and decline to take medicine because of suspicion that it is poisoned. May request foods that have not been peeled or opened, such as bananas, hard-

Provide for nutritional needs by allowing choice of food. Medicine may require injection but may be resisted less if the patient has developed trust in a staff member.

boiled eggs, and canned foods, especially if living at home or in a community facility.

Aloof, presenting an air of superiority which discourages interaction with others in the environment.	Reinforce self-esteem in honest and realistic manner. Compliment if possible on some behavior or accomplishment that has meaning to the patient to reduce isolation.

The use of drugs in treatment requires that nursing personnel be vigilant in observing and reporting changes in behavior or evidence of side effects. Signs that disturbing symptoms and behavior are diminishing and that the patient is taking more interest in others and in activities should be recorded, with description of the activity or behavior on which the judgment is based. The use of drugs combined with psychotherapy, milieu therapy, and other forms of treatment that may be prescribed, supported by quality nursing care, has as its goal the restoration of the patient to the optimum level of health possible. As in other chronic health problems, many patients who are victims of a schizophrenic disorder display symptoms, respond to treatment, and utilize resources to cope with their health problems.

Example: A young man previously hospitalized with a diagnosis of schizophrenic disorder accompanied his mother and a friend to dinner at a hotel where a nursing convention was in session. He picked up a brochure from a display table which described the symptoms of cancer. At breakfast the next morning he declined to eat saying, "I don't need food because I am dying of cancer." Asked to describe his symptoms, his answer was vague, but his manner was that of a person with a moderate degree of anxiety. Following discussion of his symptoms with a nurse who was a trusted friend, he began to eat and appeared to give up his concern.

Example: A young woman, admitted to a hospital in an acute state of confusion and suspicion, was refusing food. The nurse tasted the food to reassure the patient that it was safe. Although this did not immediately get the patient to eat, she did say to the nurse, "I'll eat if you get me a Coke to drink." The nurse, who usually carried some change in the pocket of her uniform, left the floor and went to the floor below where there was a Coke machine and bought the Coke for the patient. The patient ate her meal, gave no further problem about food or treatment, and was discharged from the hospital a few weeks later. At the Christmas season, the former patient came to the unit with a box of candy for the staff. She said that she was convinced the staff wanted her to get well when a nurse used her own money to buy her a Coca-Cola: "From that day I felt that all of you were trying to help me."

Example: A girl in her last year of high school began coming home from school and going immediately to sit beside a small fish pond in the backyard of her home. When her mother asked her why she was doing this, she replied vaguely, "I go to watch the fishes swim." Although she had not previously concerned herself with the fish, her mother was surprised but did not consider this behavior of great concern. Only when she began to get up during the night and go to the fish pond was a physician consulted. About this time the daughter became acutely disturbed and was hospitalized. Hallucinations and delusions were present. She was unable to respond in a coherent manner, even distorting the pronunciation of her name and unable to recall her home address.

Patients with schizophrenic disorders, like patients with diabetes and other chronic conditions, frequently require continuing supportive health services. Many are currently being restored to various levels of functioning. Some return to former occupations, others to personally comfortable, but reduced occupational functioning, and many return to live at home or in a supervised and sheltered environment.

In the past, many of these patients remained in state hospitals for essentially a lifetime. They often contributed to the maintenance of the hospital, performing a variety of tasks, making few if any demands, and participating minimally in recreation or socialization.

Psychopharmaceuticals combined with psychotherapy, milieu therapy, and social and rehabilitative services in current use have reduced the number of long-term patients in institutions.

AFTERCARE SERVICES

At present, some patients who are discharged in remission may not have a welcoming family to return to. They may be discharged from treatment to group homes in which they fail to share communal tasks and activities. They may wander away and survive in a state of poverty and degradation, lacking the ability and initiative to seek help. They may return to and re-enter a psychiatric hospital.

If early intervention is successful in establishing more comfortable relationships and a more rewarding life, a brief period of hospitalization and treatment combined with continuing treatment in an outpatient service may be effective in avoiding further hospitalization. The treatment plan should include the opportunity for making friends and developing interests, hobbies, or work that is satisfying. It is also important to learn that human beings are entitled to a variety of options in lifestyle and behavior. Continuing support to assist these individuals to cope with unusual stress and anxiety should be available and acceptable. Members of the family, peer-group members, and significant others can be helpful if they are informed and prepared to recognize evidence of overloads in relationships or work.

Social and recreational clubs and organizations staffed by volunteers, some of whom are mental health professionals, serve to keep the patient in contact with reality and to offer opportunities for socializing. In many areas, aftercare services are provided by community health nurses who answer the questions of the patient and family and determine if the patient on continuation of prescribed drugs is having any side effects that require further attention by the clinic or psychiatrist. The visit of a community health nurse serves a special function in association with family members in maintaining chronically ill patients in home and community.

LEARNING ACTIVITIES

1. Arrange with your instructor to participate in the nursing care of a patient admitted with a diagnosis of schizophrenic disorder. Record the behavior and conversation of the patient. If possible, talk with the person or persons who accompanied the patient to the hospital and record your conversation with them. Use direct quotes or concentrate during your conversations with the patient so that you can record the specific content and the behavior observed.
2. Request assignment to orient the patient to the unit. Record the behavior and any verbal responses to introductions and any comments on the facilities. Be especially alert to any evidence that the patient will ask questions. Take time so that the patient will not feel hurried. Be alert also that any part of the orientation appears to be disturbing or increasing anxiety, and reduce the stress by terminating the orientation, or delaying it until later, explaining to the patient that he or she must be tired and wish to relax.
3. You are assigned to provide nursing care for a patient with a schizophrenic disorder. Prepare a nursing care plan, using the nursing process:
   Assess the patient's nursing needs.
   Plan (with the patient) for action, setting time limit and goals.
   Implement the plan in collaboration with the patient to the extent feasible for the patient's participation.
   Evaluate the result (achievement of goals), and note any modification made in the original assessment, plan, and implementation.

BIBLIOGRAPHY

AMERICAN PSYCHIATRIC ASSOCIATION: *Diagnostic and Statistical Manual of Mental Disorders (DSM-III), ed 3.* The Association, Washington, DC, 1980.

BAILEY, DS AND DREYER, SO: *Therapeutic Approaches to the Care of the Mentally Ill.* FA Davis, Philadelphia, 1977.

CARTER, FM: *Psychosocial Nursing,* ed 3. Macmillan, New York, 1981.

DOONA, ME (ED): *Travelbee's Intervention in Psychiatric Nursing,* ed 2. FA Davis, Philadelphia, 1979.

EDWARDS, MS: *Psychiatric day programs: A descriptive analysis.* J Psychosoc Nurs Ment Health Serv 20:17–21, September, 1982.

GREEN, H: *I Never Promised You a Rose Garden.* Holt, Rinehart & Winston, New York, 1964.

HARRIS, AC AND MCCARTHY, K: *Mental Health Practice for Community Nurses.* Springer, New York, 1981.

HARTIGAN DEL CAMPO, EJ, CARR, CF AND CORREA, E: *Rehospitalized schizophrenics.* J Psychosoc Nurs Ment Health Serv 21:29–33, June, 1983.

LIPKIN, GB AND COHEN, RG: *Effective Approaches to Patients' Behavior,* ed 2. Springer, New York, 1980.

MODLEY, DM: *Paranoid states.* J Psychiatr Nurs 16:35–37, May, 1978.

ROBINSON, L: *Psychological Aspects of Patient Care,* ed 3. FA Davis, Philadelphia, 1976.

SAXTON, DF AND HARING, PW: *Care of Patients with Emotional Problems,* ed 3. CV Mosby, St Louis, 1979.

Film
Introduction to Psychiatric Nursing. Lippincott A/V Program, Philadelphia, 1977.

CHAPTER 10   *BORDERLINE PERSONALITY DISORDER*

Judith Morris, M.A., R.N., C.S.

LEARNING OBJECTIVES

> ***Study of this chapter should prepare the student to:***
> 1. List some of the major characteristics of the person diagnosed as having borderline personality disorder.
> 2. Give examples of manipulation.
> 3. Recognize splitting of staff and how to avoid it.
> 4. Identify own feelings when caring for the person with borderline personality disorder.
> 5. Develop a beginning plan of care for the major nursing problems associated with a patient who is diagnosed as having borderline personality disorder.

Borderline personality disorder* has received much professional attention in recent years and encompasses many diagnoses used previously, such as latent or ambulatory schizophrenia or schizophrenic character.

---

*Category from *Diagnostic and Statistical Manual of Mental Disorders (DSM-III)*, American Psychiatric Association, 1980.

CHARACTERISTICS OF BORDERLINE PERSONALITY DISORDER

The patient with borderline personality disorder has extremely unstable affect, behavior, social relationships, and self-image. The patient has short-lived, intense personal relationships, self-destructive behavior, marked shifts in moods and attitude toward reality, poor impulse control, and feelings of blankness or emptiness. The borderline disorganization of personality is characterized by impulsive behavior in areas that are often self-destructive. Although borderline patients are relatively stable emotionally, they may regress into short-term psychoses when stressed. Disturbances of consciousness are not unusual. Patients often have difficulties in school, leisure, work, and home life. Reality testing is not always entirely reliable and may be distorted depending on the response of the listener.

Borderline patients often experience difficulties in social relations, especially with sexual partners, since they lack empathy and show few feelings except for anger, anxiety, and loneliness. They are sometimes described as lacking common sense, and are said to have great potential that they seldom attain. They frequently blame others for their failures and refuse to accept responsibility for their actions. These persons are almost always intolerant of being alone, and are afraid of being abandoned by significant people in their lives. They lack the ability to gain enjoyment from everyday life and readily return to a state of dependency when faced with the need to make decisions required of adults. There is an inability to correctly interpret the subtle messages of others, and they are often tactless in their responses. They tend to view each person as either all good or all bad. This behavior is called "splitting." Borderline patients tend to assume an attitude of believing themselves someone special and deserving of extraordinary consideration by others. There is a grave lack of control of anger, and they often complain of boredom. Manipulation of others is characteristic, and they do not understand why the manipulated person becomes angry.

Manipulation, poor impulse control, splitting of staff, self-destructiveness, and regressive dependency are the behavioral hallmarks of borderline patients that must be recognized by all staff members involved in their care.

Manipulation

Examples: A 50-year-old black female with a long history of hospitalization was very adept at manipulating staff. She telephoned the unit to tell staff she had taken an overdose of her medication washed down with booze. Although her speech was clear and coherent, she was admitted to the emergency room and her stomach pumped. When no pill fragments were recovered, she admitted that she had not taken any pills and had only wanted some attention because she felt lonely. Another manipulative patient told the nurse: "The weekend was so long without you. The other nurses are nice, but you seem to be the only one who truly understands. I was lonely and felt nobody cared while you were away. I couldn't sleep and was in a panic, but no one would talk to me. Could you possibly give me your phone number? I wouldn't tell anyone and would just use it in case of emergency."

Poor Impulse Control

Examples: A patient with poor impulse control was discussing anger and the difficulty in talking about the anger with the nurse. Suddenly the patient turned and slammed the nurse's hand against the wall, resulting in two fractures of the hand. A man with borderline personality disorder went on a pass and arrived back on the unit with a strong odor of alcohol on his breath, a black eye, and multiple cuts and bruises. "What happened was Joe dared me to chug-a-lug a glass of bourbon, which I did. Then a man in the bar called me a queer so I had to fight. It wasn't my fault."

Splitting

Example: One patient was able to split staff by telling his nurse, "You help me so much more than Dr. Smith does."

Self-Destructiveness

Example: A self-destructive patient called the unit obviously intoxicated to report a suicide attempt and hung up before the staff member could respond.

Regressive Dependency

Example: A regressive, dependent patient was a 36-year-old man who had just lost his 33rd job. Instead of looking for another, his solution was to go home to his mother and "have her look after me."

NURSING CONSIDERATIONS

On admission to a psychiatric hospital, regressive behavior is often seen first. The person may "act out" in manipulative suicide attempts that must be taken seriously. The patient is usually quite angry and uses a great deal of testing behavior. Later, these patients tend to appear to become model patients. They are often elected president of the community and in general assume a helping role with other patients. During hospitalization, which should be brief, a discharge date should be set early and the patient notified. As the discharge date approaches, there may be regression and return of many of the former negative behaviors, but the date should not be changed if at all possible. The multidisciplinary treatment team should ready the patient for discharge and therapy to be maintained on an outpatient basis.

The borderline patient is extremely good at emotionally involving staff members who work with them. Staff may be split into different camps which view the patient much as the patient views them: either all good or all bad at different times, depending on whether the patient receives special treatment or has had limits set. This splitting by the patient is the reason staff members view the patient so differently and either become very angry and want to punish, or feel sympathetic and want to rescue and support the patient. Splitting is evident if staff members take sides when the behavior of the patient is being described. Nurses can detect splitting and stop it by reporting and discussing the behavior in team meetings or morning reports. It is of primary importance that staff members recognize that they are human beings with human emotions and that the borderline patient will evoke in them a full range of emotions, including anger, depression, guilt, frustration, and empathy. Having feelings does not represent a failure on the part of the staff member, but emotions and their sources must be recognized to be able to continue to work with the patient in a therapeutic manner. It is essential that each staff member discusses and resolves feelings about the borderline patient in team meetings for the multidisciplinary team to work with the patient with a consistent, unified, and therapeutic approach.

Patient's Symptoms and Behavior	*Suggested Nursing Interventions*
Poor impulse control, such as substance abuse, gambling, drinking, and overeating.	Tell the person what you see him or her doing.
	Set realistic limits, such as: "You will be in the unit at 9:00 PM or you will not attend the jazz concert Saturday evening."
	State the consequence each time a limit is broken so the patient knows what to expect.
	Tell the patient about Alcoholics Anonymous, Gamblers Anony-

mous, and Overeating Anonymous, and encourage attendance.

Teach the patient the problem-solving method (nursing process).

Discuss incidents that precipitate impulsive acting-out, and have a person come up with acceptable alternative methods of behaving.

Encourage the person to discuss feelings instead of acting in an impulsive manner.

When an incident of impulsive behavior occurs, talk with the person in a matter-of-fact way and refrain from being bossy or punitive.

Serve as a role model for behaving in a rational manner.

Encourage the patient to value improvement and not become too discouraged by a single recurrence of impulsive behavior.

When a person demonstrates handling anxiety in an appropriate manner, offer positive feedback.

Structure the schedule of activities so events have a pattern of predictability.

Physically self-damaging acts, such as suicidal gestures, self-mutilation.

All threats of a suicidal nature must be taken seriously by nursing staff, even if they are believed to be manipulative. Suicidal precautions may be required.

Maintain a physically safe environment.

Assess the lethal risk of threatened damaging acts.

Demonstrate care and concern by protecting the patient from acting on dangerous impulses.

Protect from ridicule by other patients when a suicide threat is followed by a slight scratch or cut on the wrist.

Help the patient talk about own feelings.

When something goes wrong for the patient on the ward, move at once and discuss appropriate ways to handle anxiety. If suicide attempt occurs, provide immediate first aid, such as for a cut, apply pressure; for hanging attempt, release pressure on neck, give mouth-to-mouth resuscitation or CPR as necessary.

Be aware of signs of increasing anxiety and attempt to lower the anxiety.

Sometimes incidents of self-mutilation are disguised as "accidents." Discuss what was going on with the patient prior to the "accident."

Regression-Dependency.

It may be necessary to assist the patient and gradually encourage independence.

Treat the patient as an adult. Set short-term realistic goals with the patient.

Avoid making decisions for the patient. Give positive feedback when behavior is appropriate.

Address the patient by title (Mr., Mrs., or Ms.). Do not use first name or nickname.

Discuss issues and responsibilities involved in dependent, independent, and interdependent behavior.

Encourage participation in group activities as patient progresses.

A return to regressive-dependent behavior may occur when discharge is mentioned, as the date draws near. Proceed with plans for discharge and discuss the setback in a matter-of-fact manner.

Plan for the patient to participate in multidisciplinary-treatment team meeting.

Physical complaints must be checked for a possible organic basis. Report to supervisor for appropriate referral.

Caregivers may unconsciously reinforce a patient's dependency. Staff should point out to each other behavior that is reinforcing the patient's dependency or regression.

Anger.

Discuss with the patient incidents that precipitate anger, and alternative methods of behaving.

Do not respond to anger with anger.

Redirect the anger and anxiety into constructive activities, such as occupational therapy project, exercise.

Spend time with patient when not angry.

Provide staff consistency when responding to anger.

Do not joke or tease.

Set limits prior to the destruction of property. This may involve retirement to a quiet room.

Inform patient that physical violence or verbal abuse will not be tolerated.

Use calm, nonpunishing approach.

Avoid physical contact. This may be misinterpreted as a physical assault.

Reinforce appropriate behavior.

Demonstrate the appropriate use of anger by your own behavior in situations where something has happened to anger you.

Ask the patient to talk about how anger affects relationships with others.

Walk with the patient if restless.

Select a time when the patient is not angry to discuss anger.

Be available when the patient wants to talk about angry feelings.

Assist patient in accepting responsibility for the consequences of anger.

Manipulation.

If you fail to recognize a manipulative act, accept it when co-workers tell you it has occurred.

Set firm limits that give the patient a consistent set of expectations.

Require the patient to participate in setting the limits so there is not only awareness of limits but also of the consequences when limits are broken.

Share information and care plan with multidisciplinary treatment team and with staff around the clock so that a consistent approach is used by all personnel.

Accept no gifts.

Be aware that praise and flattery are usually manipulative behaviors in persons with this disorder.

Discuss each incident of manipulation of you and others with the patient so that it is clearly seen how this affects interpersonal relationships.

Do not become discouraged when the patient makes a little progress and then slips back.

Avoid responding to manipulation with anger that may result in avoiding the person. This interrupts the therapeutic relationship.

Be matter-of-fact in your approach to the patient.

Give the patient positive feedback when he or she functions in an appropriate manner.

Loneliness, marked intolerance of being alone.

On admission, introduce the patient to the patients and staff members on the unit.

Ask the patient to tell you when feeling bored. (Boredom is a symptom of loneliness.)

Discuss leisure activities to learn something of the patient's interests.

Encourage the patient to develop consistent long-term relationships (make friends).

The patient will require counseling and supervision so not to destroy relationships with manipulative and angry behavior.

Talk with the patient about the pros and cons of having a pet on discharge. Ownership should include responsibilities involved in caring for a pet.

Discuss with the patient the wisdom of not renewing relationships with former associates who abuse alcohol.

As the patient's behavior improves, suggest attendance at group therapy.

Role-play conversations the patient might initiate with peer group to counteract peer pressure.

Structure the patient's day so there are specific times when staff will be available to talk.

LEARNING ACTIVITIES

1. Request assignments to work with a patient with a diagnosis of borderline personality disorder. Review the characteristic behaviors generally associated with patients with this diagnosis.
2. Plan with the patient a course of action that both of you believe will help the patient cope with unacceptable behavior. Set specific goals and a time limit for achievement. Review progress at intervals, and discuss limits, failures, and achievements. Be realistic in giving praise or pointing out problems.
3. Record your conversations and interactions with the patient (immediately following them to retain completeness and accuracy of content). Use the suggestions for nurse action to guide your responses to the patient.
4. Use your record of your work with the patient for discussion with team members. Seek guidance from team members to assist in evaluating your actions in response to patient behavior.

BIBLIOGRAPHY

AMERICAN PSYCHIATRIC ASSOCIATION: *Quick Reference to the Diagnostic Criteria from Diagnostic and Statistical Manual of Mental Disorders, DSM-III*. Washington, DC, The Association, 1980.

BROWN, J: *The therapeutic milieu in the treatment of patients with borderline personality disorders*. Bull Menninger Clin 45:377–394, 1981.

EVANS, FMC: *Psychosocial Nursing*. Macmillan, New York, 1971.

NURNBERG, HG AND SUH, R: *Time-limited psychotherapy of the hospitalized borderline patient*. Am J Psychother 36:82–90, 1982.

SCHULTZ, JM AND DARK, SL: *Manual of Psychiatric Nursing Care Plans*. Little, Brown & Co, Boston, 1982.

WILSON, HS AND KNEISEL, CR: *Psychiatric Nursing*. Addison-Wesley, Menlo Park, Calif, 1979.

CHAPTER 11

INTERRUPTING THE CYCLE OF CHEMICAL DEPENDENCY

M. Teresa Mullin, M.S., R.N.

LEARNING OBJECTIVES

Study of this chapter should prepare the student to:
1. Define chemical dependency.
2. Identify and describe the characteristics of chemical dependency.
3. Recognize the signs and symptoms of chemical dependency.
4. Identify nursing intervention appropriate to the chemically dependent person.

The term drug addiction is currently used in discussions of alcoholism. Alcohol is a central nervous system depressant, as are other drugs for which those who become addicted develop illnesses whose major characteristics are identical to alcoholism. Alcohol or any other drug is a substance, and some state agencies have used the term "substance abuse." Drugs that are usually abused are those that alter the mood, giving a person a feeling of euphoria (well-being) or a "high." In the treatment of alcoholism and other drug abuse, the term "chemical dependency" is being used. Alcohol and other drugs are chemicals, and those who become dependent on them suffer from the illness of *chemical dependency.* Many other mood-altering chemicals, such as Valium, Librium, and Equanil, are similar to alcohol in effect. They include those prescribed by physicians as well as illicit drugs to which a person can become addicted.

In nursing, the positive use of drugs is learned and appreciated, and it may be difficult for nurses to face the lethal and/or addictive use of drugs, especially those with mood-altering effect. This is of utmost importance owing to the synergistic effect of depressant drugs, that is, the action of each drug increases the depressant action of the others.

In 1956, the American Medical Association recognized alcoholism as a disease. In 1983, the U.S. Department of Health and Human Services identified alcoholism as the number two health problem in the United States. It affects all ages, races, creeds, sexes, and levels of social status. Ten percent of the population are afflicted, and one American family in three is affected. However, education about the illness as a primary disease is often not addressed in our schools of health care with this same magnitude. Attention is focused on alcoholism's effects, which cause other illnesses such as gastritis, hypertension, fractures and trauma from accidents, anemias, heart arrythmias, depression, pancreatitis, hepatitis, mood swings, maladjustment to adult life, cirrhosis, esophageal varices, and other diseases.

FACTS ABOUT ALCOHOL AND OTHER MOOD-ALTERING CHEMICALS

Chemical dependency may be defined as a disease in which a person is dependent on drugs either psychologically or physically, or both. The dependency follows administration of a drug on either a periodic or continuous basis.

What classifies it as a disease, and what are its characteristics? According to the World Health Organization, disease is determined by etiology (causes), predictable outcome, and specific signs and symptoms.

Etiology

The etiology of chemical dependency is still unknown. One line of thought has proposed that there is an inborn metabolic disorder. A study in Sweden (Noble, 1978) on 2000 male adoptees disclosed a meaningful correlation between diagnosed alcoholism and the biologic rather than adopted parents. A further study confirmed the finding that individuals reared apart from biologic parents were significantly more likely to have a drinking problem if their biologic rather than adoptive parents had been alcoholics

(Jellinek, 1960). A large percentage of alcoholics are children of alcoholics. This suggests that at least some part of familial risk is a genetic rather than a modeling effect. More recently, the shift has been toward cognitive functioning, such as how the individual perceives getting "high" (Turkington, 1983). More than likely, the result of research will be a multifactoral approach to etiology, as cited in Lawton (1981).

It is becoming well established that chemical dependency is a primary illness, one that is not caused by another illness. Often when a person has been depressed, it is assumed that the depression caused the misuse of mood-altering chemicals. That is not true. These chemicals are drugs that depress the central nervous system. Frequently, the *effect* of this illness, depression, is treated as the primary illness, when it is the secondary diagnosis or the secondary cause. In many groups, however, it is still socially stigmatizing for a person to be identified as being dependent on mood-altering drugs. Nevertheless, it is not caused by bad morals or lack of will power.

Predictability

Another characteristic of chemical dependency is that it is a chronic condition. There is no cure, and the final outcome often is fatal unless the disease is arrested. In alcoholism there are significant differences between men and women. For women, there is a telescopic effect; once women establish a heavy drinking pattern, they develop alcoholism more rapidly than men. There may be a greater condemnation coupled with fear of being a social outcast, and feelings of guilt, all of which contribute to the concealment of drinking (Chafetz, 1974).

Because of the already mentioned stigma, it is easy to understand that *denial* is the major symptom. Denial is like a blinder that prevents the person, and sometimes those who surround the person, from recognizing the serious consequences that are resulting from misuse of mood-altering chemicals.

Numerous defense mechanisms are used to put other persons at a distance. This is done by *blaming* and *projection:* saying that it's everyone else's fault, not mine (e.g., if someone else did more, if this happened or that happened, then I wouldn't have had to do this). It is always someone else's fault. *Rationalization* is intensified and the person always has an excuse. It might be hormonal changes, working too hard, the job, the neighborhood, or that everyone else does it, and the excuses go on ad infinitum.

Other people that are affected, but not necessarily afflicted, are spouses, siblings, and parents. Certainly the whole family becomes affected, as well as co-workers, employers, employees, and colleagues. They also can unknowingly encourage the person to stay sick longer, and become affected themselves because the blame often gets shifted to them, and they too can analyze or explain it all away.

SPECIFIC SIGNS AND SYMPTOMS

The other feature of chemical dependency is its specific signs, with a downward progression ending in death unless the illness is arrested. One symptom is an increase in drug tolerance. Paradoxically, American society today applauds this symptom with cliches such as "Hold your liquor like a man" and "Women drink but never get drunk." Social drinking and other drug abuse may be expected and encouraged not only at times of celebration, but also when feeling blue or anxious. Many eating places boast their "happy hour" extending well over 60 minutes.

Specific medical signs nurses can look for to assist in confirming the diagnosis of chemical dependency are (Fluharty, 1983):

hypertension unrelieved by antihypertensive drugs
tachycardia
hepatomegaly
red palms
elevated SGOT beyond 37
MCV (mean corpuscular volume) above 97
glycosuria
increased ketones
male feminization (enlarged breast, decreased hair distribution, decreased testosterone)
impotence
unexplained seizures
aversion to sweets
night sweating (calories turn into heat not fat)
abnormal sleep patterns
forceful heart beats

increased arrythmias
need for larger and more frequent requests for pain medication
heartburn (reflux of acid)
morning nausea
an irregular ovulatory cycle
easy gagging
abdominal cramping
agitation
anxiety
mood swings
mental confusion
organic brain syndrome
disorientation
"goose flesh"
bone aches
delirium tremens
hyperthermia
convulsions

requesting mood-altering drugs   change in pupils
by name

Obviously, any one of these signs alone would not necessarily make a diagnosis of chemical dependency.

Intervention

The downward progression of alcoholism and other drug abuse can be arrested at any time. It is not therapeutic to wait until the person has reached "bottom." Chemical dependency is like an elevator going down that can be stopped at any floor; however, it is very seldom that someone is able to push that button alone. The drug-dependent person needs someone to help. The health care worker can be a major influence on helping a person seek help. Intervention (Johnson, 1973) is helping motivate the person to get help before there are major losses in his or her life, such as family, legal, or job, or before the tragedy of the late stages of chemical dependency occurs.

Dr. Vaillant's (1983) recently published research on Harvard graduates and blue-collar workers found that, much to his astonishment, Alcoholics Anonymous is helpful and successful with alcoholics. He states that Alcoholics Anonymous is the most effective means of treating alcoholism, both for sophisticated, Harvard-educated loners, as well as for gregarious blue-collar workers. There are also similar programs for other types of chemical dependency that are patterned on Alcoholics Anonymous.

NURSING CONSIDERATIONS

Facts alone are not sufficient. The attitude that all health care personnel have about alcoholism and other drug abuse is important. The first step is to come to grips with one's feelings about personal use of mood-altering chemicals. With a positive attitude and knowledge of the previously mentioned signs, the nurse is in a strategic position to foster the intervention process. It is noteworthy that the nurse's role is one of fostering rather than performing the intervention. In this regard, it is imperative that the nurse be aware of trained professionals to either refer the patient to or assist in conducting the intervention.

The nurse should never forget the strong characteristic of denial that a chemically dependent person has. Whenever a patient lets down this barrier of denial and becomes vulnerable, the nurse's genuine care and knowledge of facts can penetrate. The nurse can be the one to push the stop button for the patient on the downward progression of chemical dependency.

Many chemically dependent persons need treatment in an environment where they face reality and learn that they have been substituting drugs for people. This illness is sometimes referred to as a disease of feelings where the person learns to stand still and feel the pain without reaching for a drug to numb the pain. Treatment facilities specific to the interruption of chemical dependency should have a program designed for families to learn as well as to express feelings about how the patient's illness has affected them.

Patient's Symptoms and Behavior	*Suggested Nursing Interventions*
On admission to a treatment unit the patient may have symptoms of acute withdrawal such as nausea, restlessness, tremors, profuse sweating, poor appetite, and sleeplessness even with sedation.	The primary aim of nursing care is to allay fears during the acute withdrawal phase.
May be disoriented and confused.	Keep under close observation.
May experience hallucinations.	Take appropriate action to diminish acute discomfort.
May be depressed and suicidal.	Providing safety may require a quiet, protective environment where the nurse's presence communicates empathy.

The complexity of chemical dependency has baffled professionals and laymen alike for years. Fortunately, the time has come when individual strands of the tangled ball of yarn have been identified and provide elements of hope and help to persons and the families of persons suffering from chemical dependency.

LEARNING ACTIVITIES

1. Discuss in class your personal attitudes and bias regarding persons with chemical dependency.
2. List the ways that you and your colleagues foster denial.

REFERENCES/BIBLIOGRAPHY

BLOCK, M: *Don't place alcohol on a pedestal.* JAMA 265:2103–2104, 1976.
CHAFETZ, M: Press conference, October, 1974.

FLUHARTY, D: *Medical signs and symptoms.* Lecture—videotape presentation, Peninsula Psychiatric Hospital, Hampton, Va, 1983.

GLATT, M: *Group therapy in alcoholism.* Br J Addict 54:21–28, 1957.

JELLINEK, EM: *The Disease Concept of Alcoholism.* College and University Press, New Haven, Conn, 1960.

JOHNSON, V: *I'll Quit Tomorrow.* Harper and Row, New York, 1973.

LAWTON, MJ: *The Role of the Rehabilitation Counselor as a Facilitative Gatekeeper for the Alcoholic and Licit Drug Abuser,* Rehabilitation Monograph Series, No. 5. Virginia Commonwealth University, Department of Rehabilitation Counseling, Richmond, Va, Summer, 1981.

NOBLE, E: *Genetic and family factors relative to alcoholism.* In NOBLE, E (ED): *Alcoholism and Health: Third Special Report to the US Congress from the Secretary of Health, Education and Welfare.* National Institute on Alcohol Abuse and Alcoholism, Rockville, Md, June, 1978, pp 57–60.

TURKINGTON, C: Cognitive deficits hold promise for prediction of alcoholism. Monitor, June, 1983, p 16.

VAILLANT, G: *The Natural History of Alcoholism.* Harvard University Press, Cambridge, Mass, 1983.

VAILLANT, G: *New insights into alcoholism.* Time, April 25, 1983, p 46.

VEREBEY, K AND BLUM, K: *Alcohol Euphoria: Possible Mediation via Endorphinergic Mechanisms.* J Psychedelic Drugs 11:305–311, 1979.

WHITE, WL: *An annotated history of the use, promotion, and prohibition of mood-altering drugs.* In *Drugs In Perspective.* National Institute on Drug Abuse, US Department of Health, Education, and Welfare, Rockville, Md, 1979.

CHAPTER 12

MANAGEMENT OF VIOLENT AND ASSAULTIVE BEHAVIOR

LEARNING OBJECTIVES

Study of this chapter should prepare the student to:
1. Define violent and assaultive behavior.
2. State some reasons why patients commit violent acts.
3. Identify possible steps staff members can take to prevent violence.
4. Describe appropriate nursing actions when violence occurs.

Linda Brown, in a paper presented in a continuing education series conducted by the Western Interstate Commission on Higher Education in Nursing, defines violent behavior as a "physical act that has as its intent infliction of physical damage on another person or on property."

Violence in the health care setting is most likely to occur when a patient feels threatened by a situation or circumstance and is convinced that there is no way to exercise control or escape the threat. Only a small percentage of mentally ill patients commit acts of violence against others. An acutely disturbed patient may respond to overcrowding, lack of privacy, or restrictions on freedom. The patient may destroy an object or attack a person who is near and who is believed to be the person denying the freedom to leave the unit or the institution.

A patient who is angry and threatening harm to others may, if preventive action is not taken at once, break a window in the lounge, placing others in danger and inflicting self-injury. An intoxicated person in the emergency room or the admissions office of a hospital has the potential for destruction of property, as well as for doing violence to others in the area. A patient experiencing auditory hallucinations or delusions of a threatening or accusatory nature may respond by an attack on another person who is considered responsible for a danger to the patient's own safety or well-being.

Example: A man who was a patient was standing in a cafeteria line, convinced that the patient ahead of him was planning to poison him. The delusion prompted the patient to pick up his tray and strike the person on the head. The patient explained that he wanted to distract the patient in front of him so the patient could not carry out the plan to drop a vial of poison in one of the trays of food. He said that he was afraid he would not be sure which tray had the poison.

Committing an act of violence or aggression against another may be a humiliating experience for a patient. The goal of nursing should be prevention. The establishment of a trusting relationship between a patient and staff members should be an initial priority. Intervention which avoids violence is therapeutic and, therefore, helpful for the patient to develop self-control.

Example: A consultant, collecting data for a study, was observing a staff member on a psychiatric unit, when the staff member got up and walked across the lounge to an aged patient who had seated himself next to another man, and begun speaking to the man in a confused, rambling manner. The staff member approached the elderly patient and asked him if he would like to go to the television lobby to watch a program. The patient willingly accompanied the staff member. When the data collector asked the staff member later what had happened, the reply was: "That patient (indicating the man to whom the elderly one had been speaking) is very tense this morning. I felt that having the elderly patient talking to him in a rambling, confused manner might cause him to have a blow-up."

Patient's Symptoms and Behavior	*Suggested Nursing Interventions*
May appear tense, fearful, and suspicious.	Observe carefully for increasing tension, and in a relaxed manner suggest an activity that the patient appears to enjoy, or a change of location, to distract the patient.
May make demands for special privileges and changes in policies or	Provide information on policies, procedures, and schedules. Discuss

schedules. Demands may be posed in presence of other patients or staff, accompanied by threats.

May be unable to respond to preventive measures, and provoke an angry response to verbal abuse of a fellow patient, attack a staff member, or engage in destruction of property.

Patient is in restraint and seclusion.

them with the patient, and post on the bulletin board. The disturbed patient needs assurance of consistency in treatment. If possible, have a "quiet room" available with explanation of its purpose and regulations for its use posted. This provides the patient opportunity for self-removal from the tension-producing environment, and helps reduce the feeling that the "quiet room" is punitive seclusion.

When intervention to avoid an act of violence fails, restraint may be required. The plan prepared for the treatment program should be initiated. A team leader, with sufficient personnel to effectively restrain the patient, should be immediately available. Staff members should remove eyeglasses and other items that might be used as weapons. Restraint should be applied quickly and quietly, with the team leader telling the patient what is being done and why.

Nursing personnel should be immediately accessible or in constant attendance, discussing the purpose of the treatment in a calm, reassuring manner. Emphasize that he or she is respected and accepted as a person, but that violence and aggression against others is unacceptable. The patient should be told that the restraint and seclusion are for personal safety until self-control is re-established.

A full description of the episode and the events leading to it, as well as a full record of the patient's behavior, responses, and conversation during the restraint and seclusion should be kept. Staff members should be alert for clues to what provoked the episode so preventive steps can be taken.

If other patients are in the area where the violent behavior occurred, the episode should be discussed with them. They need to understand the problem and the action required to safeguard the patient and others. Violent or assaultive behavior is usually a humiliating experience for the patient. Safeguarding self-respect while helping the patient understand and control violence against self and others is essential.

Nurses in community agencies are sometimes called by a family member when there is a crisis involving a disturbed member. The patient's disturbed and disturbing behavior may be an alcohol or drug abuse crisis. The nurse should obtain as much information as possible about the behavior when the request for assistance is made to make an appropriate assessment of the potential for danger to others. If the request for help suggests that violence is probable, the nursing agency will usually request that police accompany the staff member. The goal of nursing will be the establishment of a trusting relationship that successfully avoids a violent act while arrangements for hospitalization, if indicated, are completed.

LEARNING ACTIVITIES

1. Request an opportunity to participate in a nursing care plan for a patient who has a history of episodes of violence.
2. Observe the patient's behavior for clues which suggest that the patient is having a problem with self-control. Try to identify causative factors, and discuss your ideas with your instructor.
3. Review policies and procedures on the unit where patients who may commit acts of violence are being treated. Review the treatment plan and outline the actions being taken to avoid episodes of violence. Prepare a report of your study for class discussion. Include an outline of the record you would keep if assigned to help with or care for a patient who commits an assault on another patient.
4. Plan a visit to a community nursing service to inquire about experiences with violent or assaultive patients. Report what you learned to members of the class.

BIBLIOGRAPHY

BABICH, KS (ED): *Assessing Patient Violence in the Health Care Setting.* Western Interstate Commission on Higher Education in Nursing, Denver, 1981.

BAILEY, DS AND DREYER, SO: *Therapeutic Approaches to the Care of the Mentally Ill.* FA Davis, Philadelphia, 1977.

BARILE, L: *A model for teaching management of disturbed behavior.* J Psychosoc Nurs Ment Health Serv Vol 20 (No 11), November, 1982, pp 9–11.

CARTER, FM: *Psychosocial Nursing,* ed 3. Macmillan, New York, 1981.

HARRIS, AC AND MCCARTHY, K: *Mental Health Practice for Community Nurses.* Springer, New York, 1981.

MAAGDENBERG, AM: *The violent patient.* Am J Nurs Vol 83 (No 3), March, 1983, pp 402–403.

Aggressive Behavior. Psychiatric Nursing Standards. Eastern State Hospital, Williamsburg, Va, 1982, p 4.

CHAPTER 13

CHILDREN AND YOUTH AT HIGH RISK FOR EMOTIONAL PROBLEMS

Patricia Nottingham Robinson, M.A., R.N., C.C.N.A.

LEARNING OBJECTIVES

Study of this chapter should prepare the student to:

1. Describe the impact of the formative years and parental relationships on the development of healthy attitudes in children.
2. Define the term *high-risk children.*
3. Describe the dynamics concerning children who are from divorced families, children whose parents have had psychiatric hospitalization, children of alcoholics, and children who have been abused.
4. Identify nursing goals and interventions that will be supportive in understanding the stresses of high-risk children.
5. Explore the importance of an ongoing personal assessment so that the response of staff to high-risk children will be productive and therapeutic.
6. Define primary, secondary, and tertiary prevention.

A variety of traumatic experiences makes today's child and family more vulnerable. It is important for nurses to recognize the dynamics of high-risk children and their families. The nurse must be able to recognize signs of stress in a child and take an active part in treatment planning. Listening, recording, empathizing, and communicating are important activities in recognizing and understanding the needs of high-risk children.

THE CHILD AND THE FAMILY

The relationships with the family, especially the parents, are the first human relationships in a child's life. The family cultivates, molds, and refines the personality. The experiences of a child during the first 12 years are most important. The child begins to observe the environment during the infant stage, begins to explore that environment at toddler stage, and reacts to the environment at latency, preadolescent, and adolescent stages. Developing healthy interpersonal relationships is a strong foundation for any child. The family provides a "practice area" for this phase of development, with parents as consistent teachers. If a child receives reasonable amounts of love, warmth, and acceptance from the parents, relationships will be viewed with ease, comfort, and self-assurance in later life. Rejection and indifference during a child's early development can lead to rebellious acts and other disturbing behavior. As teachers, parents must offer the child understanding and set limits to teach the necessity of having self-discipline. This is important so that the child will have a successful view of standards, rules, and principles. This will also help the child in adult life to become an effective limit setter for his or her own children. But parents must set limits with love and caring. Failure to do so may contribute to antisocial behavior in later years. Consistent love and support of parents allows a child opportunity for achievement in all stages of development, and enhances self-esteem.

Members of a family have many stresses placed on them. These stresses make children in the family vulnerable to traumatic situations. All families must deal with economic, social, and psychologic factors. Many mothers today are working outside the home. One fourth of the mothers of infants and toddlers, one third of the mothers of 3- to 5-year-olds, and one half of the mothers of 6- to 17-year-olds are employed. This may have a significant impact on these children because they have less contact with their parents during the early years. The child receives substitute care from other relatives, day-care agencies, or friends. The readiness to acquire independent skills may be developed prior to the ability to handle them. This often places extra stress on the child. Many children who were accustomed to one parent living in the home while the other parent worked have had to adjust quickly to two working parents.

Social factors that affect a child within the family are changes in family structure and lifestyles. In 1974 the divorce rate increased 135 percent, with more than a million children below 18 whose parents were divorced. Divorce lends itself to reorganization of living arrangements, formation of second families, and the need for children to deal with separations and losses. When this occurs during the child's early years, the child's alliances become divided between parents, and stability of development becomes altered. Parents naturally become involved in their own problems and life stresses. As a result, psychologic factors affect the child within the family. Parents who are disturbed by major life events may become psychologically disturbed, and turn to alcoholism, divorce, or child abuse. The impact of these maladjustment patterns on the children may go unnoticed.

It is important for parents under stress to see clearly its effects and set specific goals and interventions to reduce or soften the impact on their children. These children are to be considered at high risk for the development of emotional problems. *High-risk children* are those who during their formative years are faced with traumatic experiences that may create unhealthy coping mechanisms in their later years. They become vulnerable to experience maladaptive behaviors themselves because of their immaturity. Parents become less and less capable, during those traumatic experiences, to be the teachers that are needed in the child's development.

In a recent article in the *New York Times,* Winn (1983) reports on the change in society's attitude about childhood. Instead of the "age of protection," she relates that we are now in the "age of preparation." New beliefs have transformed children into knowing about the adult world earlier. This is not planned, but evolved out of need. For examples, she cites substance abuse prevalence, divorce, two-career families, premature experimentation with adultlike habits, and women's liberation. With these changes, health care professionals must be prepared to support these children.

CHILDREN OF DIVORCED PARENTS

Family loyalties are strong in families that are intact and functional. Divorce represents, in a child's eyes, the break-up of family loyalty and the need to choose between two parents whom the child cares about deeply. Divorce represents constant wishful thinking of wanting the two parents to get back together, and many children hold onto this hope until late adolescent years.

During a *predivorce period,* the home generally experiences chaotic living patterns, stress and emotional confrontations and, in some cases, physical violence. If this is the case, we find that children may begin to experience somatic symptoms characterized by nervous twitches, loss or gain of weight, appetite changes, ulcers, and vomiting, which are signals that the child has been affected. Behavioral difficulties may be characterized by anger, anxiety, guilt, grief, and/or regression, as discussed below.

Anger

"Why does this have to happen to me? It's unfair. Daddy, you were supposed to stay with us forever!" These were the words of a 9-year-old boy named Chucky whose parents were divorced. Many times children cannot discriminate between what is best for either parent, and thus focus on anger. Many children become irritable and use anger as a defense, even though they may feel sad. Younger children experience temper tantrums or become over-obedient. In dealing with angry feelings there may be blaming of a parent, especially of the mother if the father leaves the house. They look at the parent who leaves the house as being the victim, and the parent who stays as being the initiator, regardless of circumstances.

Anxiety

Children worry and may ask "Who is going to support us?" They see the economic structure as changing, especially if Dad leaves the house, and Mother is not working. Many feel that their world is turned upside down. Coupled with anxiety is fear of abandonment, the fear whether divorce will happen to them. Younger children look at divorce through fantasy and dreams as a result of anxiety. Many children may fear that they themselves will be asked to leave and worry about who will take care of them.

Guilt

These feelings are most paramount with preschool and young school-age children. They often feel that they were the cause of the separation, and may say "If I had been a better child, this would not have happened." Adolescents often retreat into thoughts such as "If I had stayed home more and washed the dishes more or had not argued with my parents, this would not have happened."

Grief

Children view divorce as a loss in which they go through stages of grieving similar to loss by death. Many children may respond with periods of depression, withdrawn behavior, or a display of disturbing behavior. Regardless of the behavior, a child's vulnerability is heightened during this period.

Regression
Preschool children may, during the divorce period, revert to infantile play, bed-wetting, and a need for participation in the rituals of the family. Security toys or blankets may be constant companions. Older children may begin to have difficulty with interpersonal relationships, may display acting-out behavior, excessive preoccupation, premature independence from the family, and verbalization of being ashamed about the divorce.

A Story From a Child's Point of View

I'm 13 years old, and my parents got a divorce. When I first heard about it, I felt that it was all my fault. I felt confused and isolated. I dreamed that it would not happen, and on my recent 13th birthday, I wished that this bad dream would go away. My parents did not tell me together—only my mom, who said that Daddy was leaving the house and staying in an apartment. I felt an emptiness because I was used to Dad's stuff being around, and I didn't know how we were going to pay the bills. Mom didn't work. Grandma said that Mom and Dad don't love each other, but they still love me. If they loved me, then this would not have happened. Grandma, Grandpa, and Mom all said that they will be close to me. The only thing that hurts is knowing that my dad, whom I love, will not be with us anymore. I feel sad.—*Mary, age 13*

CHILDREN OF PSYCHIATRIC PARENTS

When a parent is hospitalized for psychiatric treatment, it places an added stress on the family. This particular high-risk group of children has received little attention. One can readily speculate that prior to the hospitalization of the sick parent, the environment that the child lived in was chaotic. During the hospitalization of the parent, the child may wonder what the parent is doing, and becomes concerned. "Will this happen again?" The major areas of concern are discussed below.

Separation crisis leading to deprivation of care
When hospitalization occurs, one can anticipate disruptions in child-care arrangements, disruptions in health care maintenance, and possible separation from school, community, and the parent who remains in the house-

hold. It is not uncommon to have temporary caretakers, such as a grand-mother or a good neighbor. Rice, Ekdahl, and Miller (1971) point out that the assuming of a child's care by relatives is often uncertain because of the length of the parent's hospitalization. This may involve sending children to other homes or separating siblings. It is not uncommon to have temporary caretakers who are frightened by psychiatric disturbances and avoid in-volvement. For these children, dealing with the trauma of separation and caretakers' attitudes heightens their feelings of fear, rejection, and anxiety. Older siblings play a significant role in substituting as a parent, but this also puts a strain on the child.

Differences in mother's and father's hospitalization
Regardless of it being the mother or father who is hospitalized, this does not eliminate feelings of worry or anxiety. With more mothers employed now, the impact becomes greater because parents of dual-career families are ab-sent during the day, and this situation lends itself to dependence on tempo-rary caretakers. Moreover, studies have shown (Sussex, Gassmon, and Raf-fel, 1963) that prolonged absence of mothering without consistent substitution deprives children of parent-child binding.

Involvement in disturbances of a hospitalized parent
The involvement of children in the symptomatology of a parent's distur-bance can range from minor incidents to upsetting incidents. Many chil-dren who witness bizarre and inappropriate behavior of a parent may show bewilderment, fright, and sadness. Research has shown that disorders of schizophrenia and other psychoses predispose children to maladaptive coping mechanisms. In extreme cases, children may witness or be involved in delusions or hallucinations prior to the hospitalization of the parent. Many children have reported having to set limits on a parent's behavior until hospitalization. Other situations that are not this extreme have a direct impact on children. Visual observation of the disturbed parent creates sus-ceptibility for a child to internalize the distress. The gradual deterioration of a home environment may cause a child to see himself or herself as the reason for conflicts. Many times, the parent who is supporting the identified parent (spouse) may forget the child's concern, failing to realize that misrep-resentations or distortions may be occurring.

A Story From a Child's Point of View

I am 12 years old. I saw my mother sleeping quietly one morning. Daddy had gone to work, and I had the responsibility of fixing cereal for my two younger brothers and sisters. But 10 AM came, and Mom did not wake up. I tried to shake her, but she wouldn't move. I then picked up the phone and dialed 911 for emergency. They took Mom to a hospital for people who have problems. You see my mom took pills because she was sad. I became sad and scared to visit her because I thought she was going to die. I feel relieved, but this is not the first time this has happened. I remember two other times when Dad took her to the hospital. I hope she gets better. Going to the hospital and visiting her helps, but I'm afraid it will happen again.—*Sheila, age 12*

Additional Themes That Concern the Children

1. Embarrassment to tell anyone.
2. What can I do to change?
3. I'm behind in schoolwork because of worry.
4. I'm tired of all those babysitters.
5. Will it happen again?
6. Should I behave differently?
7. My stomach gets upset every time I visit the hospital.
8. I can't sleep anymore.
9. What does the nurse do?
10. I feel lonely and sad.
11. Will it happen to me?

CHILDREN OF ALCOHOLICS

In the United States, there are somewhere from 28 to 34 million people who have been reared in the home of an alcoholic. Twelve to 15 million teenagers under the age of 18 are living with at least one alcoholic parent (Black, 1982). Research points out that the children of alcoholics are affected not only by the alcoholic parent, but by the parent who is nonalcoholic. Alcoholism is a multigenerational disease that predisposes a child to become a high risk for alcoholism as well as marriage to an alcoholic, or to develop patterns of maladaptive behaviors. According to Black (1982), some children take on one of the following roles in the family.

The Responsible One
As we have seen in the children of psychiatric parents, these children also take on the overwhelming task of adult behavior at an early age. This causes them to become preoccupied with being self-reliant and controlling. They fail to enjoy their childhood as other children do.

The Adjuster
These children learn to separate themselves from stresses in the family. They may appear reserved, withdrawn, and aloof at situations that would normally be a cause for reaction. In their world, they have not been able to handle the parent's drinking. They give up on their wishes that life may be better and dismiss the belief that they may have some control over their own lives.

The Placater
These children take care of the practicing alcoholic parent, the other parent and siblings, but do not have time to take care of themselves. They have come to believe that their feelings and concerns are not important, but they strive to make the family less unhealthy.

The feelings of sadness, guilt, shame, and confusion are hard for children to deal with. The basic reaction is to deny that alcoholism is happening and continue to fit into one of the roles described.

Traditional roles also play a significant factor in the family. If the alcoholic is male, he is accepted or tolerated more than a female. With mothers who are alcoholic, behavioral and emotional problems may be due to interruptions in the mother-child bond (Cork, 1969). Children also see that the parent's drinking is a reflection that something is wrong in their household and consequently may conclude "I am a bad person."

These children are greatly influenced by alcoholism; they see parents as role models and may imitate their behaviors. They risk becoming alcoholics themselves.

A Story From a Child's Point of View

I am 15 years old, and a child of an alcoholic. I had to be the adjuster in my family because my father had numerous personality changes as a result of alcohol. When he was drunk, he was rigid, and argumentative with my mom. He wouldn't care about me, my homework, or me as a person. When he wasn't drunk, we got almost anything we asked for. It was difficult to adjust to these changes, but after several times I learned to adjust for survival. I knew what kind of attitude to have when he was sober, and when he was drunk, I stayed out of his way. My fear is that one day I may not adjust in time, which will make my dad mad, and then I'll feel bad.— Chrissy, age 15

CHILDREN WHO ARE ABUSED

The Child Abuse and Treatment Act of 1973 states: "Child abuse and neglect means the physical and mental injury, sexual abuse, negligent treatment or maltreatment of the child under age of eighteen by a person who is responsible for the child's welfare under circumstances which indicate that the child's health or welfare is harmed or threatened." Since this bill was passed, all states have passed legislation that requires health care professionals to report suspected cases of abuse to local protective services courts. Child abuse has placed conscious awareness on the caregiver in mental health settings. Child abuse in many instances is unspoken or evidences are not clear-cut, while other forms have physical implications. The types of abuse are discussed below.

Physical Abuse
Physical abuse involves voluntary, purposeful acts of bodily harm.

> *Examples:* Hitting, kicking, slapping, pushing victims out of windows onto floors, tying to beds or cribs, whipping, hitting with ropes or belts.

Physical Neglect
This is not a result of poverty. It is voluntarily and purposefully depriving children of physical, emotional, nutritional, and medical-care needs.

> *Examples:* Lack of provision of food, hygienic needs, immunizations, and for protection from falls, and from swallowing harmful liquids. Broken bones discovered on x-rays, buccal-nasal lesions, finger deformation, and damage to nasal membrane.

Emotional Abuse
Emotional abuse is the deliberate verbalization of harsh words, name calling, and so forth that causes the individual to feel worthless, unwanted, or unloved.

> *Examples:* Name calling, using profanity, and never praising but offering constant negative comments.

Emotional Neglect
This involves lack of providing a nurturing environment that affords the child recognition, love, praise, security, and the feeling of belonging. The

young infant and child are susceptible to this because of consequences of inadequate mothering.

Examples: Failure to thrive in young infants, lack of human contact, ignoring, and not providing appropriate toys to aid in growth and development.

Sexual Abuse

Sexual abuse is violent and nonviolent sexual activity or contact with a child. It includes incest, which is intimate sexual physical contact by family members. Sexual abuse includes not only sexual intercourse by arousal activities, but the failure of an adult to report these activities or to intervene for the well-being of the child.

Examples: Sexual intercourse, fondling genitals, oral sex, and anal intercourse.

The diagnosis of child abuse is often difficult because of the child's fear of verbalizing what has happened. Generally, the child's behavior is withdrawn and passive, and little attention from parents is sought on admission. Some children may exhibit "grabbing reaction" as a direct result of wanting to belong. Many times, the child appears lethargic and presents a blunt affect. Enuresis, encopresis, refusal to eat, and vomiting may also occur. Many children may be resistant at first to helping a caregiver for fear of reprisal and a need to protect the abusive parent. Some may be wary of physical contact with adults and may cry excessively or become silent during treatment in the emergency room or other treatment facilities. Some children will not engage in eye contact with a caregiver or may exhibit a vacant frozen stare.

Abusive parents are under stress and are unable to cope with external or internal stressors; thereby, they manage their daily living ineffectively. Many parents have been abused themselves, so that parental abuse has a generational derivative. Specifically, abuse in families is the result of parents not being properly parented and so having never learned parenting. Abuse episodes can also occur after changes in financial status, the loss of a job, or a change in the living situation, and from lack of knowledge of the developmental stages of children and adolescents. Many times abuse is associated with not being able to handle stress from illness in the family, whether this is mental or physical dysfunctioning. Abusive parents are usually suspicious and distrustful of others. This keeps them sometimes from being able to share problems, as well as from being able to release tension. Tension is thus focused and ventilated within the family.

Morris and co-workers (1974) have identified four types of abusive parent: (1) the *undercontrolled parent*, that is, the impulse-ridden parent who is angry and blames the child for family problems; (2) the *overcontrolled parent*, who feels punishment, even if it results in injury, is necessary to correct a child's behavior; (3) the *fantasy-prone parent*, who responds to unrealities of the inner world rather than the real world and the child; (4) the *guilt-ridden parent*, who is disturbed about the abusive treatment of the child.

A Story From a Child's Point of View

I'm 10 years old and live with my mom and three brothers. My name is Maria. Daddy left us 6 months ago, and we have not heard from him. I often remember the fighting and fussing Mom and Dad did all of the time. I thought that things would be better since Mom and Dad split up. But Mom became sad and was upset all the time. Then she began to fuss at us, and hit me real hard in my stomach. She gets mad at me for no reason. I thought I was good, and I do try extra special. It happened so much I ran away to Grandma's. I didn't tell her what happened, but I didn't want Mom to hit me anymore. What do you do when Mom screams and hollers at you for no reason? I'm scared!—*Maria, age 10*

IMPORTANCE OF NURSING INVOLVEMENT

Children at high risk for emotional disorders are part of every health care delivery system. Many of these children are hospitalized for various physical or emotional problems that are not labeled "child of divorced parents," "child of psychiatric parent," "child of alcoholic parent," or "abused child." However, as the helping professional works with children and adolescents, it is important to undertake the following steps to achieve the nursing process:

1. Take an active part in the multidisciplinary team conferences, and see yourself as a viable team member.
2. Review charts and look at familial history, whether it is of the child or family member, in the hospital or outpatient setting.
3. When it is identified that the child has high-risk factors, learn the dynamics of such children, as stated in this chapter.
4. Identify each member of the family with regard to marriages and divorces.

5. Identify if there are any financial stressors in the family, such as loss of job, death, alcoholism, mental illness, and the like.
6. Provide a supportive climate in your therapeutic setting to allow the child and family to ventilate feelings.
7. Participate in any supportive interventions or programs that may occur in the treatment setting.
8. Recognize the importance of teaching as a fundamental basis for allowing children and their families to develop healthy coping mechanisms.
9. Participate actively in family programs utilizing group skills.
10. Participate in discharge or follow-up planning from various health care settings.
11. Record your observations accurately.

PERSONAL ASSESSMENT

Working with children of high-risk families is not an easy task. One's beliefs, values, traditions, and life experiences influence the care that these children and families receive. It is important to be committed to serve these patients without prejudices. It is also possible that attitudes, thoughts, and feelings occur without an awareness of their effect on the patient. Society's values have a tremendous influence on the staff member. Review the following questions, therefore, with yourself, your peers, and your supervisor. Begin to share openly your feelings. Allow yourself to think through the questions and receive the feedback of your peers and supervisors.

Children of Divorce

1. How do I feel about divorce, especially when the children are young?
2. What is my reaction to the family's discord, and the dissolution of the family?
3. If I am from a family where divorce occurred, do the readings from the family history relate to me?
4. Do I feel frustrated and angry with a family member (father or mother) who leaves the home where children are involved?
5. Do I fix blame on any given party?

Children of Psychiatric Parents

1. How do I feel about society's stigma on mental illness, and can I see it from a child's perspective?

2. Do I feel that a child will automatically acquire dysfunctional behaviors because one or both parents couldn't cope?
3. After reading a family history and listening to its impact as verbalized by the children or adolescents of the family, is it my feeling that it could have been prevented?

Children of Alcoholics

1. Has there been alcoholism in my family, and if so, how do I feel about it? What were my family's beliefs about alcoholism?
2. Do I portray sympathy or empathy as I assess the child's needs.
3. What are my feelings toward alcoholic parents, and how do I relate to them? Is my communication clear, open, and honest?

Children Who Are Abused

1. Do I feel disgusted or repulsed at the child's home situation?
2. Can I relate to some of the home situations, and if so, do I feel this will be an asset or hindrance in developing therapeutic communications?
3. Do I feel that the family's situation is hopeless?
4. Do I find myself more anxious, or more fearful, in the child's presence?

PREVENTION

It is important for nurses and other caregivers to recognize levels of prevention as they work with high-risk children. Caplan (1961) has been a pioneer in prevention and early intervention. His approach has been supported by public health workers. Three levels of prevention are considered in providing support to high-risk children. All three levels can occur in an inpatient setting as well as an outpatient setting.

Primary Prevention

Primary prevention is aimed at reducing the incidence of mental disorder in children by strengthening the capacity of children and their parents to understand and tolerate stresses. Programs emphasize the promotion of healthy families. Children at risk need to be identified so that preventive services or treatment planning can be initiated. Nurses have an important role in all programs.

Programs:

1. Classes for families on child development.
2. Prenatal classes for new parents.

3. To prevent child abuse: child advocate on pediatric units specializing in family assessment; various parent education classes conducted by churches, schools, and other facilities.

Secondary Prevention

Secondary prevention aims at reducing the prevalence of mental disorders through early case finding and effective treatment. Early case finding helps in early referral to appropriate health services.

Programs: Team conferences, nursing intervention, family counseling, short-term hospitalization, and maintenance of therapeutic environment. Children and adolescents who are hospitalized will benefit from these programs.

Tertiary Prevention

Tertiary prevention aims to reduce long-term disability and assist patients in returning to a home environment. Nurses in community services have an important role in rehabilitation that facilitates productive ways of coping in home and community.

Programs: Follow-up home visits, discharge-planning conferences, and continued parental teaching.

LEARNING ACTIVITIES

1. Visit an agency and talk to health professionals who work with children at high risk, as described in this chapter. After your visit, plan a team conference and discuss your observations, using the participant observer form on the next page. You may inquire about appointments to visit children and adolescents in inpatient settings, outpatient community mental health agencies, or child guidance clinics.
2. Using the nursing process as a guide, identify approaches to use in working with high-risk children and their families.

REFERENCES/BIBLIOGRAPHY

ANTHONY, J AND KOUPERNIK, C: *The Child in His Family: Children at Psychiatric Risk.* John Wiley & Sons, New York, 1974.

BARRETT, C: *Child Abuse* (unpublished manuscript), Family Development Association, 1982.

BLACK, C: *It Will Never Happen To Me.* MAC Book Dept, Denver, 1982.

CAPLAN, G: *Prevention of Mental Disorders in Children.* Basic Books, New York, 1961.

PARTICIPANT OBSERVER EXPERIENCE

Agency _____ Date _____

Type of Programs Available

Helping Professional's Role

What I Learned

Questions for Class Discussion

Student: _____

CHESS, S AND THOMAS, A: *Annual Progress in Child Psychiatry and Child Development.* Brunner/Mazel, New York, 1981 and 1982.

CORK, MR: *The Forgotten Children.* Addictive Research Foundation, Toronto, Canada, 1969.

GABEL, S: *Behavioral Problems in Childhood.* Grune & Stratton, New York, 1981.

GARDNER, R: *The Parents Book About Divorce.* Bantam Books, New York, 1979.

HABER, J, ET AL: *Comprehensive Psychiatric Nursing.* McGraw-Hill, New York, 1982, pp 883–1012.

KJERVIK, D: *The contemporary American family: Romanticism vs reality.* J Psychosoc Nurs Ment Health Serv 20(3):9–12, March, 1982.

MORRIS, M, ET AL: *Toward prevention of child abuse.* Child Today 4(2), 1974.

PAVENSTEDT, E AND BERNARD, V: *Crises of Family Disorganization: Programs to Soften Their Impact on Children.* Human Sciences Press, New York, 1971.

RICE, E, EKDAHL, M, AND MILLER, L: *Children of Mentally Ill Parents.* Behavioral Publications, New York, 1971.

ROBINSON, P: *Children of psychiatric parents* (unpublished manuscript), 1983.

ROFES, E: *The Kids' Book of Divorce: By, for & About Kids.* Random House, New York, 1982.

SUSSEX, GASSMON, AND RAFFEL: *Adjustment of children with psychiatric mothers in the home.* Am J Orthopsychiatry 33:829–852, 1963.

WINN, M: *The loss of childhood.* New York Times, May, 1983.

CHAPTER 14   # MENTAL HEALTH PROBLEMS OF CHILDREN AND YOUTH

Faye Gary Harris, Ed.D., R.N.

LEARNING OBJECTIVES

Study of this chapter should prepare the student to:
1. Describe depression in young children and identify appropriate nursing interventions.
2. Describe the disturbed and disturbing child and identify appropriate nursing interventions.
3. Identify the signs and symptoms seen in the adolescent at suicide risk and list appropriate nursing interventions.
4. Describe anorexia nervosa and bulimia and list some suggestions for nursing intervention.

DEPRESSION IN YOUNG CHILDREN

The *depressed child* is usually sad and lonely. The child feels a sense of isolation and loneliness. The loneliness transmits thoughts that the interpersonal situation is void of any possibility of these feelings being lessened. The child engages in solitary play, thus becoming further removed from interpersonal situations. Hopelessness and helplessness dominate waking hours.

When depression is suspected, the child's history for "losses" must be evaluated. Then an accurate history should seek to elicit a response that presents itself as (1) a meaningful relationship with another, (2) real and imagined feelings of loss of the significant other, (3) rebellion against the loss, (4) mourning for the lost person, and (5) detachment and estrangement. Thus, children of divorces, parental death, illness, or prolonged separation are high-risk children.

The nurse or other professionals examining the child should check for antecedent behaviors to depression. A checklist might include: (1) school failure, (2) drug and alcohol usage, (3) phobic-type behaviors, (4) pervasive anger, (5) rebellion against authority, (6) threats or actual runaway behaviors, and (7) complaints of headaches, stomachache, or other somatic-type complaints.

Patient's Symptoms and Behavior	*Suggested Nursing Interventions*
Child feels sad, lonely, and isolated.	Have the child describe the feelings being experienced in the current situation.
Child may have thoughts of being unworthy of attention, love, and caring.	Listen with interest and look for specific and real reasons for these thoughts. Assess appropriately whether the thoughts have a cause-effect relationship in reality.
Child complains of physical problems, e.g., headaches, stomachaches, and lack of appetite.	Ask for physical examination to rule out organic difficulties. Determine how long these physical problems may have persisted.
	Look for onset of physical problems that might correspond with perceived or real losses.
	Set up a contractual arrangement for eating if food or liquid intake is a problem.
	Provide "presence" for the child when child is experiencing somatic complaints. Inquire about the nature, characteristics, duration, and intensity of the physical complaint.
	Use play therapy as a method of encouraging the child to act out symptoms, thus the conversation can be guided to focus on anger, resent-

The child has a mental picture of how life will be after death. Are there ideas of suicide involved? Are there happy or sad feelings associated with thoughts of "life after death"?

ment, and rage concerning the loss of a love object.

Determine the following concerning life after death:

- Are these thoughts and feelings with the child continuously?
- Are thoughts and feelings of being united with loved ones present?
- Are there plans for joining the loved ones?
  - Suicidal plans should be explored with the child. Playing with puppets and other types of dolls is useful. Drawing and finger painting are other helpful methods of inducing expression.

The child has fears, thoughts, and feeling of loss, isolation, separation because of physical illness (acute or chronic), impending surgery, or other intrusive procedures.

Discuss with the child the necessity of specific procedures. Explain, through drawings and other modes, the functions of specific organs and organ systems, the impending procedure, and the likely outcome. Provide opportunities for child to cry, experience outbursts, and articulate anger, rage, hopelessness, and helplessness. Strategize to provide a base in reality by which child can "check out" facts and fantasies regarding impending or ongoing situations.

Child or family has fears about physical/emotional care of child.

Provide health care information concerning the complete care of the child's posthospitalization or postprocedure to the family members. Information for use, should there be an emergency, is of extreme importance. Be specific and provide names, addresses, and telephone numbers to cover a 24-hour period.

Fears, apprehension, anger, and hopelessness may prevent child from seeking peer relationship.

Establish a trusting relationship with child. Engineer situations in which child can excel. Explore motor activities if there are strengths in this area. Gradually program one child, then two children, to play with the depressed child. Do not reject child; a staff person who "likes" the child

Child has difficulty sleeping.

might be a prerequisite for determining who the therapist should be.

Provide a favorite staff person to be with child during time leading up to sleep states. Staff might sing child's favorite song. Make up words that feature the worthiness of the child (the strengths of the child, e.g., an excellent bicycle rider, superb reader, pretty eyes, etc.). Record sleep behaviors.

Child has ideas and plans to involve in runaway behaviors or drugs (now or later); discusses keen interest in sex; manifests temper tantrums, etc.

Child discusses fears of getting close to other children and adults.

Document all content and explore with child plans to implement these ideas.

Explore with child *alternative* ways of expressing resentment, rejection, and rage. Some possibilities include:

- Try to invest in another person.
- Trust another in order to experience the joy and warmth of caring for another/another caring for child.
- Involve self in activities in an effort to learn how to sublimate feelings and thoughts, thus creating opportunities for mastery now and in later life.
- Ventilate and express thoughts and feelings to others and gradually expose "pent up" resentments, distortions, and perceptions.
- Provide content to others (adult) who are useful in planning and discussing healthy alternatives to depression.

Patient's motor activities might be retarded.

State that child is worth waiting for, that clinician feels that child is deserving of time and human investment. Compliment child when clinician sees improvements. Provide opportunities for eye contact. Provide opportunities for body contacts; children respond to tactile stimulation. (Be sure that this approach is not contraindicated.)

Child pulls hair, mutilates parts of body, or refuses food.

Careful observation and documentation of, and specific interventions for, safety are appropriate if child is engaging in any of these behaviors. Weight and height charts should be kept on all children.

Patient's Personal Hygiene and Appearance

The encopretic and enuretic child might have residue on body. Smells will increase feelings of unworthiness and self-depreciation.

Child neglects personal appearance because of feelings of unworthiness. Looks disheveled and indifferent from lack of sleep. Has feelings and thoughts that no one cares for child.

Suggested Nursing Interventions

Check child's body for soil. Assist in shower, bath, and other activities that will clean child. Apply perfume or cologne to child's body for pleasure.

One assigned member works with child and talks with child while assisting with dress, personal grooming, etc. Prepare/assist child in preparation of clothing that is attractive, appropriately fitted, and clean. Clothing and dress habits should reflect the weather conditions.

Patient's Treatment and Activities

Family assessment for purpose of establishing the utility of further family counseling or therapy.

Suggested Nursing Interventions

The clinician must be versed in family dynamics from both practical and theoretical points of view.
- Establish how family feels about the child.
- Gather information concerning family's perception of when difficulties began; assess the role functions of family members; document and clarify the family's perceptions of the child's role within the family (e.g., Was the child always different? Is this child the family member destined to be sick?)
- Clarify what the family expects from treatment.

Group therapy provides the child with opportunities to develop relationships under the "watchful eye" of the therapist.

The group process should be safe for the child. Interactions among peers should be encouraged. The therapist can plan and implement numerous techniques that enhance self-esteem for the patient and other group

members. For example:
- The stroking game: everyone takes turns and talks about the good attributes of the patient.
- Trust-talk: Share difficult situations with group. Here the therapist guides the group toward clarification of distortions, perceptions, facts, values, etc. Exploring alternative methods of dealing with the complexities of the specific situation is the aim.

Individual therapy.

Individual therapy may be concomitant with group or family therapy. The therapist should remember that these new relationships might be the foundations for all future interpersonal relationships.

Chemotherapy.

The clinician must be aware of specific medications, side effects, and contraindications. Any untoward signs must be reported to nursing and medical personnel immediately.

THE DISTURBED AND THE DISTURBING CHILD

The *disturbed child* can generally be categorized as one who might be experiencing internal disorganization of perception, thought, reality testing, judgment, and a sense of self that assists in separating the child from the external world. These children might be disinterested in the environment. Their affects are flat, and their expressions frequently bland and sterile. Speech is expressionless and monotonous. However, these children are quiet, self-contained in their pathologies, and do not interrupt the environmental milieu. Mothers, teachers, and community workers view such children as different but cooperative, obedient, and self-entertaining. Some people consider these children "ideal" because of their self-containing, self-entertaining, withdrawn, and isolation tendencies. They make no demands on the environment and, therefore, are not as likely to receive attention, referral, and treatment. Examples of such conditions might be childhood schizophrenia, childhood depression, degenerative disease of the central nervous system, endocrine disorders, obsessive-compulsive neurosis (depending on the degree), withdrawn reactions, and a myriad of other behaviors.

The *disturbing child* has a tendency to be disruptive and to provoke authority figures to the extent that methods of control are required. The behavior requires immediate attention and limit-setting from persons in the environment. Peer group members respond to these children with ambivalence: the ambivalence ranges from fright, fear, and feelings of helplessness to elation, vicarious satisfaction because of the defiance of authority, and fleeting feelings of security and safety brought about through identification with this peer group. Examples of health problems that cause these conditions might include hyperactive children, brain-damaged children, substance abuse populations, and hypomania.

The following categorization will provide a general schema within which to classify children as disturbed or disturbing. This schema includes a list of behaviors and descriptive differentiating content useful when working with these two classifications of children in a variety of settings, for example, the home, the school, the community, and the hospital.

The Disturbed Child

SYMPTOMS AND BEHAVIOR

Motor Behaviors

A marked decrease in motor movements and activities.

A lessened interest in the environment.

Close observations might reveal subtle or even blatant movements and behaviors that are self-contained.

Special mannerisms, speech, eye focusing, and other ritualistic-type behaviors might be involved.

Emotional detachment and preoccupation with internal thoughts and stimuli prevent any focusing and concentrating on the external environment.

An inability to follow goal-directed activities; an impoverished thought process that would hinder any goal-directed activities.

No interest or concern for the external environment; thus, no demands are placed on the environment.

Activities may be automated, that is, a few habits that are essential for institutional living may be learned, internalized, and executed in an automated fashion. For example, child enters a classroom, gets books, goes to seat, and remains there—quiet and nondisruptive—for several hours.

Internal thought processes might include hallucinations, delusions, or vivid wish-fulfilling mental pictures that satisfy the child's needs and interests that the external environment cannot satisfy.

In the home, such a child might be seen as one who plays alone very well; may be perceived by the mother or parents as being an extraordinarily "good child" who does not interrupt the mother.

Long hours might be spent in bed, bedroom, or in the designated play area involved in private thought process that tends to be nonresponsive to the external environment. Thought processes can range from hallucinations and delusions to illusions and/or an active fantasy life. Some characteristics of these thought processes will be discussed in the section below on symptoms and behavior.

In summary, the disturbed child, frequently quiet and withdrawn, and therefore not disruptive to the environment may, if observed, manifest the following behaviors and conversations:

Motor behavior will reveal a lack of zest, vigor, and spontaneity. The child might remain in a rigid body posture and in a rigid and deliberate manner. All movement of body extremities may be deliberate, forced, and lack spontaneity. The child may experience occasional outbursts of feelings and thoughts.

Special mannerisms and rituals may accompany certain tasks. These rituals are considered to be extremely important to the child and serve as a method of control over the environment.

Conversations may be disjointed and difficult to follow. They might include content about the child's rich fantasy life and/or developing delusional system. Words may have a special meaning to the child that are different from the usual interpretation, thus making communications with others strained and extremely difficult.

Hallucinations

Auditory hallucinations involve hearing voices in the head that (a) tell the child to perform certain acts and (b) provide a running dialogue concerning the behavior and thoughts occurring within the child as they transpire.

Tactile hallucinations involve the child's feeling contact (though false) being made with skin.

Olfactory hallucinations include those false thoughts that certain aromas and odors are in the atmosphere.

Kinesthetic hallucinations are false sensations about the body's being in certain positions and postures.

The nurse must remember that hallucinations are real experiences to the child, though they have no base in reality. These experiences might result in the following behaviors: preoccupied, withdrawn, socially isolated, inappropriate affect, bizarre motor movements, interrupted speech, and so on. Finally, hallucinations are triggered by internal stimuli and do not require external activities to act as an impetus.

Delusions

Delusions are false beliefs and thoughts that the child experiences. These false thoughts and beliefs do have some relationship to reality, though the content might be grossly distorted. In other words, there is a "kernel of truth" in all delusional experiences. Some characteristics of delusions include:

Delusions that the child's thoughts and feelings are being controlled by some outside system, person, or force.

A belief (delusion) that thoughts are being broadcasted to others in the environment through some elaborate system.

Delusions about the total body being ill, or a specific body system being afflicted or ill. Conversely, the child might have thoughts about the body having extraordinary powers and capabilities.

Delusions may also involve religious content, as well as beliefs and thoughts that the child might vanish or be obliterated.

The nurse has the arduous task of separating and differentiating a rich and overdeveloped fantasy system from a true delusional system. Delusional systems may not be present in younger children (ages three to five).

PERSONAL HYGIENE AND APPEARANCE

Parents, teachers, and nursing personnel must be taught to observe for sluggish eliminatory habits, weight loss, bed-wetting, and evidence of further withdrawal from interpersonal relationships.

All persons who have contact with the child should observe for reactions to certain "bodily sensation" that might be precipitated by external or internal stimuli, for example, hallucinations or environmental activities.

The child should be kept clean and well groomed. Bodily contact should be gauged by age-appropriate behavior on the part of the parents, teachers, and mental health personnel.

Interpersonal communication should be encouraged in any setting and during any task that the child and an "other" might be involved in.

The Disturbing Child

The disturbing child is disruptive in the home, the school, and the community. This disturbing phenomenon may be the result of organic, social, cultural, and other forces.

SYMPTOMS AND BEHAVIOR

Frequent disruptions of activities and conversations of others in the home, school, and community.

Snatching toys or objects from peers and smaller children, and inappropriately grinning and remarking about this feat.

In school, the child might be observed as having continuous difficulties in "taking turns" in a social setting; thus, peers are usually angry and nonsupportive of this child.

School failure is a symptom of deeper disturbances. The inattention to directions from the teacher, frequently overlayed with poor academic skills, forces the child to create other (the child's own) priorities.

Difficulty in sitting still for any period of time. In other words, the child is considered "fidgety," as well as disruptive.

Threats to one's peers of physical harm might be noticeable.

Threats and the exertion of physical harm to parents and other adults and children.

Verbal assaults accompanied by mimicking bodily movements and excitability. The target person can be anyone who attempts to set limits with the child, for example, teacher, parents, and mental health personnel.

Pervasive negativistic attitudes and behaviors toward parents and other authority figures.

The destruction of property and vandalism might be impulsive behaviors, or they might be well thought out and carefully calculated.

Lying, and placing the blame on others (peers or adults) make it difficult for the child to establish permanent ties with anyone. As a result, the child's behaviors are reinforced simply because of the lack of appropriate intervention by someone in the environment.

The child might have been disturbing earlier in life, but more disruptive and disturbing features tend to peak postpubertally (about 11 years upward).

The child usually has a record of truancy from school.

The child feels alone and isolated. The ability to establish and maintain relationships is very poor. In later years, the child might begin to identify with a gang and develop a degree of solidarity with this group.

Projects onto others those thoughts and feelings about the self that cannot be tolerated and are considered alien to the self (ego).

Fantasizes about the "great controls" that are exercised over others.

Thought content might, under close observation, reveal specific themes, patterns, and fantasies in the thought processes.

There may be (in some cases) thought disorders (see previous sections on hallucinations and delusions) that accompany these thought patterns.

When the child expresses thought content in a social context (about parents, teachers, and clinicians), it frequently is demeaning, disruptive, and debasing. There is more evidence, however, that the child does not trust, respect, or rely on the integrity of others for the purpose of getting assistance in meeting some basic needs.

In some children, the behavioral modes are expressive of thoughts and feelings *without* the accompaniment of language and speech. The child may "act out" rather than "talk out" a particular problematic situation.

Can plan activities (deviant) with some degree of accuracy and reality testing. These internal thoughts are usually not shared with others, especially adults.

In some children, thoughts of how to "conquer and control" interpersonal situations are of paramount importance. These children can become obsessed with these thought patterns. However, they seldom translate their inner thoughts into a communication mode.

The thoughts and feelings of disturbing children are directed toward activities, to the exclusion of peer interaction, except in instances in which peers can bring some type of immediate gratification to these children.

Because of the disturbing nature of these children, they are avoided, isolated, separated, and alienated from peers, teachers, and clinicians. The parents, nevertheless, are never free of the effects these children have on them.

In the severe form of disturbing behaviors, the "conscience" or superego may be undeveloped or underdeveloped. Thus, no guilt or remorse accompanies these disturbing acts. As a result, without appropriate intervention, these behaviors will continue and probably increase and require major control.

PERSONAL HYGIENE AND APPEARANCE

Diet should be carefully monitored because of this age of development.
Bath facilities should be readily available.
Clothing should be clean and styles should be appropriate to age and culture.
Hair care should be provided, and it should reflect the child's age and cultural orientation.

Treatment

Treatment for the disturbed child and the disturbing child includes:

Group therapy	Behavior therapy
Individual therapy	Sports therapy
Storytelling therapy	Milieu therapy
Art therapy	Hospitalization for intensive
Relaxation therapy	milieu-management
Family therapy	Psychotropic medication

The intervening person must, when working with children from different cultures, socioeconomic statuses, and religious groups, be careful about the clinical inferences, statements, and the conclusions when participating in the total treatment process. Frequently, consultation with someone from a similar culture or background or with a professional is recommended. Finally, the "disturbed child" is a deeply troubled child, who may have at one time manifested behaviors similar to those behaviors identified in the "disturbing child." Perhaps, then, a second level of illness is evidenced in the disturbing child; the first-level illness might be conceptualized as being those clusters of behaviors, affect, and thought processes identified in the "disturbing" phenomenon.

Mental health care providers, on the other hand, often react to these two classifications of children quite differently. For an example, the frequently nonintrusive nature of the "disturbed child" does not necessarily infringe on the rights of others regardless of the setting (that is, home, school, and community) because of its self-contained though detrimental nature. The disturbing child, however, retaliates and disrupts homeostasis within the milieu. Their behaviors are frequently met with disgust, disdain, and helplessness.

Because of the triaging to institutions, enmeshment with the legal system, coordination of services by welfare departments, and other factors such children, in spite of blatant symptoms, do not receive adequate mental health services. It is understandable, then, to expect the Report to the President from the President's Commission on Mental Illness to have identified troubled children as a population that should receive priority in the mental health delivery system in the projected years.

THE ADOLESCENT AT SUICIDE RISK

Adolescence is probably one of the least defined areas of growth and development. Interest in adolescents by psychiatric/mental health nurses has recently begun to surface. This group, however, has presented mental health workers with perplexing problems for generations.

Adolescence, as defined by the American Psychiatric Association, is a chronologic period beginning with the physical and emotional processes leading to sexual and psychosocial maturity and ending at an ill-defined time when the individual achieves independence and social productivity. This span includes changes in behaviors, thinking, physical growth, and patterns of relation, as well as interest in the human body, new roles, and a series of continuous trial behaviors.

The normal adolescent is so "turbulent" and many times transient in mood and thoughts that this period is considered extremely difficult for the adolescent and the family. Consequently, abnormal adolescence has traditionally been considered difficult to diagnose, treat, and rehabilitate. For example, a young person might vacillate from loneliness and despair to enthusiasm, elation, or euphoria in a very brief period.

The suicidal adolescent, however, is a particular syndrome that warrants immediate attention from the clinician. This section will present materials for understanding, treating, and managing the suicidal adolescent. Here, suicide is the outstanding clinical problem. It should be remembered, however, that suicide can occur, for example, in normal individuals, schizophrenics, those with depressive reactions, crises, and so on. This approach should be helpful in the assessment and treatment of all diagnostic groups.

The clinician must consider that 15 to 25 percent of adolescent suicides

occur among the schizophrenic population of adolescents. An expert diag-
nostician might be sought for a differential diagnosis, and clarification of
one or several pathological syndromes occurring at once can be made.

Patient's Symptoms and Behavior

(Early signs and symptoms while person may/may not be in the hospital).
During mental status examination (see Chapter 4), seek information concerning suicides or attempted suicides in the family—remote and recent.

Does the person live with
- Both natural parents?
- A step parent? (Which one?)
- Have there been long periods of separation and alienation between adolescent and one or both parents?

The financial status of the family is/is not stable. How severe are the problems?

Family conflicts within the family that are severe and harsh, over a period of time.

Alcoholism and drug abuse in the family by one or more parent(s).

Severe and/or chronic illness experienced by the adolescent.

Behaviors that are signs of increased turmoil in adolescence include:
- Continuous and excessive argumentation and fighting with parents.
- Running away from home or continually threatening to run away.
- Heavy use of alcohol or other chemical substances.
- Increased sexual activity.
- Severe lability in moods.
- Severe concern about body and how others see (what they think of) it.

Suggested Nursing Interventions

Converse with person about feelings and thoughts concerning parent's suicide or any attempts. Elicit from the person the method habitually used for responding to stress, e.g., sleeping, alcohol intake, crying, seeking advice, thinking things through.

Explore the family relations that person experiences. Pay particular attention to feelings, fantasies, rage, dislikes, respect for which family member. Help person identify ways used to handle these feelings.

List any difficulty with finances that affects the person. Identify if patient is seen as causing the problem.

Discuss and list family conflicts that the patient perceives, and connect the way in which conflicts affect the patient.

The nurse should have a historical perspective about attitudes and behaviors before hospitalization. These seven areas should be explored with the patient.

Observe and document all behaviors of mood swings, conversations concerning running away, concerns about the body, and thoughts about academic functions.

- Variance in academic achievement.

Behaviors and conversations that indicate seriousness of attempt include depressive behavior that manifests itself through neglect of body and sad facial expression.

Comments about life after death are always to be explored.

Elicit verbal expressions of disappointments, losses, and extreme anger directed toward *what* significant person? Identify that person, the role function, e.g., mother—at home or away from home; girl/boyfriend—Who is dissolving the relationship?, etc.

Listen and elicit other information about previous attempts and the thoughts and feelings the patient expresses concerning them:

- Are these attempts attention getting?
- Is suicidal attempt a familial behavior?
- Is punishment of a significant other a goal? Is there another way to accomplish this goal?

The staff should evaluate the following behaviors for severity of attempt and plan nursing care accordingly.

- Degree of isolation of the patient on the ward; the conversation that claims no or few other person(s) in patient's environs.
- Did the patient communicate to anyone the intent to commit suicide before the act?
- Was the suicidal act well planned? Was the planned act lethal or superficial?
- Does the patient speak openly about joy of communicating with a dead person after patient is dead?
- Is the content of hopelessness and helplessness about life in its current state? Does the patient feel that failure is inevitable?

Recognize that suicide among adolescents is a major cause of death and therefore remove from the patient's environs all contraband, e.g., razors, belts, knives, etc.

The patient should be placed close to the nurses' station for intensive observation.

Or, an "intensive care" room should be used until severe depression and suicidal ideation abate in intensity.

Use TV monitor in room of suicidal patient to provide continuous surveillance of patient.

Or, assign special nursing personnel to be with patient at all times. The 1:1 ratio is ideal for this type of patient because it provides continuous opportunities for patient to express:

- Hostilities
- Disappointments
- Disillusionment
- Losses (very important)
- The future (oriented toward life, death, indifference, etc.)

This content is essential when planning for continuous therapy.

Food intake might need to be monitored with some patients.

Reality testing should be the focus in the nursing staff and may include:

- Perceptions of what a current situation is.
- Discussion about changing, manipulating, altering a situation.
- Feelings and thoughts that are within a person vis-a-vis the thoughts, feelings, and actions of significant others.
- Perceiving an external event accurately in terms of its severity, permanence, and total impact on the patient and others.
- A search for alternative methods of dealing with the situation, e.g.,

- Ask patient about a suicide note.
- Is the planned method of suicide bizarre?
  - Gun
  - A ritualistic ceremony
  - Pills
  - Contraband (knives, belts, razors)
- Assess the patient's ideas, thoughts, feelings concerning responsibility for own life, the desire to improve the quality of life, and the responsibility for beginning positive action.

replacement, sublimation, talking things out, etc.

Read the content of suicide note, extracting the names of significant others mentioned. Is there an issue of:
- Loss?
- Deprivation?
- A final irreversible situation?

The staff must structure the entire ward for the patient's safety. Some possibilities might include:
- Restricting visitors to unit (parts of unit).
- Locking (temporarily) all doors to unit.
- Padding walls in patient's room.
- A 1:1 (patient:staff) ratio.

Patient's Personal Hygiene and Appearance

In depressive state elimination might be irregular.

Mouth care and skin care will require special attention.

Patients sometimes experience heightened acuity to internal body.

Suggested Nursing Interventions

Encourage fluid intake, diet roughage. Monitor toilet activities.

Encourage and assist patient to take responsibility for personal hygiene (the beginning of the responsibility concept for own life).

Provide adequate make-up and toiletries for female patients and male patients (perfume, cologne, etc.).

Encourage/assist patient to dress up, look good.

Provide support, positive reinforcement, and directed conversation.

Report somatic complaints to physician.

Provide for an adequate exercise program
- On ward, patient can walk with staff.
- When well enough, patient can leave ward with staff and go for long walks (conversation, behavior, spoken concerns might be monitored).

Patient's Treatment

Individual therapy.

Suggested Nursing Interventions

Establish initial rapport and trust.

Understand the dynamics of the suicide.

Focus on self-esteem and responsibility for self.

Direct conversations toward seeking alternative behaviors to suicide
- Finding replacements for losses.
- Seeking other methods of receiving need satisfaction.

Group therapy with other adolescents and young adults.

Arrange milieu where patients can have eye contact with group members.

Be supportive and noninterpretive with patient.

Encourage sharing of feelings, thoughts, and habits.

Problem-solving, reality testing, and decision-making are overall functions of the group.

Clarification and detailed elaboration of situations involving a specific other are essential in the group process. Immediate feedback and reinforcement are primary functions of the therapists.

Family therapy may be indicated when the turmoil and suicide are outgrowths of family disturbances.

Family therapy treats the family unit and does not, initially, treat the identified suicidal patient.

Roles, values, expectations, communication patterns, and individual family needs are explored and improved on in these sessions.

EATING DISORDERS

Anorexia Nervosa in Young Women

The term *anorexia nervosa* is used to describe a syndrome that implies pubertal emaciation in young pre-pubertal and pubertal girls. This population of patients has a heightened interest in food, but they *refuse* to eat. In fact, their interest in food is considered obsessive in nature. The desire to remain slim is the factor that motivates them to abstain from eating.

As the person continues to refuse food, the body grows thinner and thinner. Many patients will try to heighten their activities for the purpose of increasing the metabolic output that burns up body fat. The nurse must remember that the patient's goal is to lose weight. The underlying conflict rests in the fact that the girls do *not* wish to grow up and be women. Their fears of sexual maturity within their environment are too threatening to allow maturation to continue. Contemporary American views about diet, slimness, and attractiveness certainly put into motion somatic and eating problems that become methods of expressing conflicts. Within the social environment, the patient is astute enough to manufacture rules, regulations, and philosophical positions that provide a framework within which she can place a well-thought-out intellectual rationalization about her unconventional habits.

Bulimia in Young Women

Bulimia differs in its characteristic behavior from anorexia nervosa, but presents the same symptoms and behaviors of a serious eating disorder. The disorder is more common in young women than in adolescent males. The person with bulimia engages in binge eating, usually in secret. Large amounts of high calorie sweets are eaten, followed by self-induced vomiting. Efforts to control eating may alternate between fasting and overeating. Occasional periods of normal eating patterns occur, but the pattern of fasting to lose weight and binge eating is likely to persist over long periods. The depression and sense of poor self-image is similar to that seen in anorexia nervosa.

Patient's Symptoms and Behavior	*Suggested Nursing Interventions*
Thoughts of fears of the impending future. A thought process that dictates that slimness is the only acceptable alternative in the environment.	The nurse must be concerned with nutritional intake and output: • Record food and liquid intake. • Record vomiting, spitting up, etc. • Record physical activities. • Record menstruation.
A thought system that cannot be expressed openly, but only indirectly, for fear of reprisals and rejection in the environment.	The nurse must work with a variety of professional staff, e.g., pediatricians, psychiatrists, nutritionists.
Fears spontaneous expressions of emotions and at same time fears verbal retaliation from significant others in the environment.	Plan situations whereby the patient can meet situations that require decisions; assist the patient in the decision-making process; encourage the expression of thoughts of fears,

Thoughts and feelings of disgust about basic body functions concerning the alimentary canal (eating, digestion, defecation, urination, etc.). Thoughts of being of normal physical stature indicate body image disturbance; while patient actually thinks that weight and height are within normal proportions, the reality is that patient is starving self.

Feelings of rejection since infancy are deeply buried in the unconscious.

Active physical programming induced by the patient may be of concern to the staff. Ambivalence is frequently expressed in the patient's behaviors and conversations: "I promised my father that I would gain weight, but he did not notice the two pounds I gained. Why bother?"

Identify a sequence of pre-anorexia behaviors; focus on patient's perceptions of family roles and activities. Ask patient to be specific.

resentment, rejection, and uncertainty that accompany the decision-making process.

Discuss thoughts and feelings concerning the body functions, specifically body image, menstruation, female sex characteristics. Devise specific socialization opportunities for the patient to communicate with members of the opposite sex. Do not force the patient to eat; assign one nurse per shift to work with the patient. In addition, a nurse therapist can be a primary therapist.

Discuss and plan for the exploration of specific ego defense mechanisms that might be useful to the patient when experiencing frustrations, existential fears.

Monitor physical exercise; sometimes patients exhaust themselves. Discuss with the patient her wish to remain slim and the reasons that growing up is painful, and help patient to select other methods of dealing with anxieties.

Check patient's caloric intake, and continue to monitor vomitus, elimination, etc.

Discuss with patient feelings and thoughts concerning family members' feelings and behaviors toward her. Identify areas of difficulty in the family communication patterns. Here are some examples:

- Mother and patient relationship.
- Mother's role within the family.
- Mother's interests and hobbies.
- Family's expectation of the patient.
- Father's role within the family.
- The decision-making process that occurs within the family.
- Identify patient's relationship with:
  - Mother.
  - Father.
  - Siblings.

Patient fears rejection and disapproval; any attempt to comply with external demand is extremely threatening and thus requires immediate recognition.

The family reacts to the patient's condition by burying hatchets and joining forces in times of crisis.

Patient's Personal Hygiene and Appearance

Large dresses and clothing are worn to disguise body image.

Skin turgor and tone might be poor.

Grooming habits might be neglected.

Sluggish eating habits result in constipation and weight loss.

Patient might refuse food, thus continuing to lose weight.

Patient's Treatment and Activities

In thoughts, feelings, conversations, and appearance, the anorexia patient appears to flirt with destiny by playing games with her body by withholding food substance.

- The communication patterns within the family relative to:
  - Sexual expressions.
  - Methods of expressing feelings of aggression, resentment, and rage.
  - Patterns, expectations, and reinforcement behaviors.

Using incremental steps toward achievements is an excellent therapeutic approach.

When there are positive changes in the patient, the staff should expect to see changes in the family system. These changes may be healthy or pathological. Notice changes in content that patient verbally expresses.

Suggested Nursing Interventions

Weigh patient daily and keep records of daily weight.

Monitor and record the types of activities that the patient engages in.

Be alert to dehydration, constipation, dizziness, and fatigue.

Continually discuss the fears of weight gain with the patient; manage not to dwell on food intake but the consequences of weight gain. Continue to identify:
- Conflictual areas.
- Recurrent themes.
- Relationships with significant others in the family setting.

Suggested Nursing Interventions

Bring to the patient's attention that caloric intake is necessary.
- The staff can prepare a caloric intake protocol.
- An elimination sheet should accompany the protocol.
- The entire treatment team decides on a weight that the patient must

achieve before discharge.

The staff must be aware of the rationale for these interventions that are used primarily in life-threatening situations; be consistent in assisting in these modalities; and understand the specific nursing care associated with the treatment.

Patient shows a dull mental status that does not allow adequate integration of a "sense of reality" with the realities of an existing physical state—anorexia.

The nursing staff must be careful not to recreate a milieu similar to the family milieu that the patient experienced at home.

- Evaluate methods by which staff communicate.
- Be aware of themes that can be extracted from the patient's conversations.
- Observe how patient relates to members of the opposite sex on the ward, e.g., staff, patients, etc.
- Instruct staff not to be highly critical of the patient; instead, encourage and support freedom of expression, ventilation of hostilities, anger, fear, and resentment.

Special therapies ordered by the psychiatrist and the pediatrician may require special action by the nursing staff:

- Electric shock therapy.
- Tube feeding.
- Hormone therapy.
- Chemotherapy.

Provide interpersonal situations whereby the patient can make decisions without hostile reprisals being a consequence.

- Autonomy in daily activities on the ward.
- Express likes and dislikes about food.
- Discuss her body, e.g., appearance, feelings of threat, dislikes, amazements, power.
- Discuss/ventilate thoughts and feelings concerning the "eating experience" (expect content that indicates that eating is a bestial and primitive act that should be avoided).
- Provide opportunities for the patient to discuss fantasies, daydreams, night dreams, and futuristic thinking with the staff. Record themes that recur in all these activities.

Treatment

INDIVIDUAL THERAPY

The development of a trusting relationship is essential but difficult. The staff must be ever so careful not to respond to the patient with aggression, hostility, and resentment.

GROUP THERAPY

The development of more effective communications can be introduced in individual therapy and reinforced in group therapy. This method of therapy can (1) help the patient identify areas of distortion in thinking, (2) aid in the instillation of hope for the future, (3) reinforce the idea that others suffer and struggle too, and (4) assist in the identification of intrapsychic conflicts.

FAMILY THERAPY

Family therapy is an excellent therapeutic mode that helps the patient and family members clarify such concepts as: (1) perceptions of the identified patient, (2) expectations/lack of expectations of the identified patient, and (3) family members' modes of communicating with the patient, for example, hostility, resentment, rejection, and indifference.

BEHAVIOR THERAPY

Perhaps this is the most popular treatment for anorexia nervosa. This approach includes the establishment of specific operant consequences, that is, positive reinforcement or punishment, depending on weight gain or weight loss. For example, for every pound gained, the patient will earn 10 tokens; for a five-pound gain the patient will earn 50 tokens or a 30-minute visit with a significant staff person.

Operant reinforcement can be set up to provide (1) shaping of behaviors by the behavior therapist and (2) introduction of reinforcers such as television viewing, walks with staff, and so forth into the eating program.

Specific therapies, in addition to milieu therapy, should yield goals and objectives in treatment. An ongoing assessment of the patient's progress is essential. This assessment should involve all members of the treatment team.

LEARNING ACTIVITIES

1. Request assignment to either work with or observe a child psychiatric nurse who is providing care to:
   A depressed child
   A disturbed and/or disturbing child
   An adolescent at suicide risk
   A teenager suffering anorexia nervosa or bulimia.
2. Record your observations and any participation for a class discussion. Use the following form.

PARTICIPANT OBSERVER REPORT

Name of Patient _____ Date _____
Treatment Program _____
Observation:

Participation:

What I learned:

Questions I have:

BIBLIOGRAPHY

Depression in Young Children:
FREUD, A: *Normality and Pathology in Childhood: Assessments of Development.* International Universities Press, New York, 1965.

FREUD, A AND BURLINGHAM, D: *War and Children.* International Universities Press, New York, 1943.

FREUD, A AND DANN, S: *An Experiment in Group Upbringing.* In EISSLER, R, ET AL (EDS): *The Psychoanalytic Study of the Child, vol 6.* International Universities Press, New York, 1951.

FRISCH, A: *Depression.* In JOSEPHSON, M AND PORTER, R (EDS): *Handbook of Childhood Psychopathology.* Jason Aronson, New York, 1979.

HARRIS, F: *A psychiatric nursing experience with a troubled child living in the community.* Perspect Psychiatr Care 5:87, 1968.

HARRIS, F AND WILSON, L: *The Depressed Child.* In SNIDER, J (ED): *Blackinston's Handbook for Nurses.* McGraw-Hill, New York, 1979.

SCHULTERBRANDT, J AND RASKIN, A (EDS): *Depression in Childhood: Diagnosis, Treatment, and Conceptual Models.* Raven Press, New York, 1977.

The Disturbed and the Disturbing Child:

AICHORN, A: *Wayward Youth.* The Viking Press, New York, 1925.

AMERICAN PSYCHIATRIC ASSOCIATION: *Diagnostic and Statistical Manual of Mental Disorders (DSM-III).* The Association, Washington, DC, 1980.

ERIKSON, E: *Childhood and Society.* WW Norton, New York, 1963.

HALL, C AND LINDZEY, G: *Theories of Personality: Primary Sources and Research.* John Wiley & Sons, New York, 1970.

HARRIS, F AND BESSENT, H: *The Triad: A Predictive Syndrome of Adult Crimes.* Unpublished manuscript, 1978.

HARRIS, F AND WILSON, L: *Mental Health Problems in Children.* In SNIDER, J (ED): *McGraw-Hill Handbook of Clinical Nursing.* McGraw-Hill, New York, 1979.

LEWIS, M: *Clinical Aspects of Child Development.* Lea & Febiger, Philadelphia, 1973.

LONG, N, MORSE, W, AND NEWMAN, R: *Conflict in the Classroom.* Wadsworth, Belmont, Calif, 1971.

RUESCH, J: *Therapeutic Communication.* WW Norton, New York, 1961.

STRAKER, N: *Impulse and Conduct Disorders.* In JOSEPHSON, M AND PORTER, R (EDS): *Clinician's Handbook of Childhood Psychopathology.* Jason Aronson, New York, 1979.

WEEKS, E AND MACK, J: *The Child.* In NICHOLI, AM (ED): *The Harvard Guide to Modern Psychiatry.* The Belknap Press, Cambridge, Mass, 1978.

WINNICOTT, DW: *The Piggle: An Account of the Psychoanalytic Treatment of a Little Girl.* International Universities Press, New York, 1977.

The Adolescent at Suicide Risk:

AMERICAN PSYCHIATRIC ASSOCIATION TASK FORCE ON NOMENCLATURE AND STATISTICS: *Diagnostic and Statistical Manual of Mental Disorders (DSM-III)*. The Association, Washington, DC, 1980.

ANTHONY, EJ: *The reactions of adults to adolescents and their behavior.* In CAPLAN, G AND LEBOVICI, S (EDS): *Adolescence: Psychosocial Perspectives.* Basic Books, New York, 1969.

BALLAK, L, HURVICH, M, AND GEDIMEN, H: *Ego Functions in Schizophrenics, Neurotics, and Normals.* John Wiley & Sons, New York, 1973.

ERIKSON, EH: *Identity: Youth and Crisis.* WW Norton, New York, 1968.

FINCH, SM AND POZNANSKI, EO: *Adolescent Suicide.* Charles C Thomas, Springfield, Ill, 1971.

HARRIS, F AND FREGLY, M: *An adolescent's struggle for independence.* In FAGAN, D (ED): *Nursing in Child Psychiatry.* CV Mosby, St Louis, 1973.

NICHOLI, AM: *The adolescent.* In NICHOLI, AM (ED): *The Harvard Guide to Modern Psychiatry.* The Belknap Press, Cambridge, Mass, 1978.

ROBERTS, S: *Behavioral Concepts and Nursing throughout the Life Span.* Prentice-Hall, Englewood Cliffs, NJ, 1978.

Eating Disorders:

BOCKAR, JA: *Primer for the Nonmedical Psychotherapist.* Spectrum Publications, New York, 1976.

CONRAD, A: *The attitude toward food.* Am J Orthopsychiatry, July, 1937.

ERICKSON, MT: *Child Psychopathology,* ed 2. Prentice-Hall, Englewood Cliffs, NJ, 1982.

FREUD, A: *Normality and Pathology in Childhood.* International Universities Press, New York, 1965.

HOLLANDER, F, ET AL: *The Regulation of Hunger and Appetite.* Ann NY Acad Sci 63:47, 1955.

PALAZZOLI, MS: *Self-Starvation.* Jason Aronson, New York, 1974.

ROBERTS, S: *Behavioral Concepts and Nursing throughout the Life Span.* Prentice-Hall, Englewood Cliffs, NJ, 1978.

STUNKARD, A AND SURWIT, R: Behavioral treatment of the eating disorders. In LEITENBURG, H (ED): *Handbook of Behavior Modification and Behavior Therapy.* Prentice-Hall, Englewood Cliffs, NJ, 1976.

CHAPTER 15

MENTAL HEALTH AND MENTAL ILLNESS OF THE ELDERLY

LEARNING OBJECTIVES

Study of this chapter should prepare the student to:

1. State the number of people over 65 years of age in the United States and the percentage who are in institutions.
2. Identify the essential information required to evaluate the health of an elderly person.
3. List some activities of mentally healthy elderly persons. Identify health and other support services needed by elderly persons who wish to remain in their homes.
4. List the activities and services available to protect and maintain the quality of life of elderly infirm and mentally impaired individuals.
5. Describe the health-promoting activities that nurses can use to assist elderly patients and their families to cope with illness and loss.
6. Describe an activity program designed to sustain the quality of life for elderly infirm patients.

There are approximately 26,000,000 people in the United States over 65 years of age. They are a diverse group in lifestyle, socio-economic status, and in their views of aging and way of reacting to aging. The number of ethnic and nationality groups lends additional variation to their needs for, and use of, health services.

One fourth of the 26,000,000 individuals over 65 in the United States are in nursing homes, state hospitals, other health care facilities, or have multiple health impairments requiring special health care. Others are living at home. A substantial number of them are living in poverty and precarious conditions of health.

The annual cost of health care for the elderly in the United States, including those living at home, averages more than $1,688 per person. Even for many of those living in comfortable homes and continuing a variety of activities, the cost of health care frequently taxes their economic resources severely. They generally must cope with more chronic ailments than younger persons. Depression is common, especially when changes occur in physical conditions, when there is loss of a friend or loved one, or when there is a perceived need for a move that threatens their sense of position in the family or community.

Planning health care for the elderly should include individuals and groups, as well as members of the families to the extent it is possible. Individuals should be encouraged to voice their opinions, concerns, and wishes, even if, in the final decision, these cannot always be honored. *Communication*, to be useful, must be *shared and understood* by each person involved.

Example: An elderly widow living with her daughter and family became ill and required hospitalization. En route to the hospital, the daughter told her mother she felt that she had not been giving her mother proper attention because she was busy with her children and husband, so when she was ready to leave the hospital she would take her mother to a "nice nursing home" where she would receive proper care. Her mother did not comment. She was a model patient in the hospital until her physician told her that she had made great progress and should tell her daughter that she could go home the next day.

The evening nurse (3–11 PM), reporting to the night nurse at 11 PM, said, "I don't know what has happened to Mrs. _____ . She has changed completely. By actual count, she has had her light on 23 times since 3 PM, asking for only minor services and not admitting any change or complaints. She has had sleeping medicine, but is not asleep. You may have a busy night."

In a few minutes the patient had her light on for attention. The night nurse responded to her request to lower the window a few inches, then lingered by the bed saying, "You're usually asleep when I come on duty. Is something bothering you?"

The patient began to cry and express a feeling of abandonment. For her, her daughter's plan for a "nice nursing home where she would receive proper care" was unacceptable, but she was reluctant to discuss it with her daughter. She felt that being sent to a nursing home meant that her daughter did not wish to have her continue living with her and her family. The daughter thought of her suggestion as improving the care of her mother. The night nurse reported to the morning staff saying, "After we agreed that this could be discussed with her daughter the next day, the patient went to sleep."

Planning appropriate health services to the elderly requires a complete and *accurate appraisal of the mental and physical condition* of each individual. The health services should be designed to include education to prevent, whenever possible, development of diseases of the elderly. Early intervention and effective treatment of illnesses, and continuing support and supervision to maintain an optimum level of health is not only desirable, but economical. Realistic planning for aging should really begin early in life and continue throughout the adult years to ensure a lifestyle that promotes health. The elderly should be able to enjoy the rewards of their earlier accomplishments.

THE MENTALLY HEALTHY ELDERLY

The shorthand definition of mental health, "a zest for living," is being acted out continuously by an increasing number of individuals in the aging population. Many elderly persons lead interesting and productive lives. They form groups and engage in a variety of social, educational, and cultural activities, as well as domestic and foreign travel. They put in many hours as volunteers in community agencies and other community activities. They own and manage businesses, are elected to public offices, and serve as professional consultants to institutions, agencies, and industries. Many continue to live in long-established homes; others in condominiums and apartments to which they have retired to reduce costs in keeping with retirement income as well as the responsibilities associated with the extensive maintenance work on a house. Many members of this group are coping satisfactorily with such chronic ailments as arthritis and diabetes, as well as other chronic conditions. They schedule their physician, dentist, and personal service appointments and maintain positive rewarding relationships with their friends and family. They retain enthusiasm, enjoying involvement with others. They are an increasingly vocal and effective group in public affairs.

For some elderly persons, activity and involvement in later life follows the lifetime pattern of an outgoing, warm, and friendly personality. For others, the "zest for living" that they now display may be related to a change of circumstances which frees them to enjoy roles and relationships not possible earlier. Still others have acquired this enthusiasm and resourcefulness in their later years, demonstrating the potential for change and adaptation possible by the elderly and challenging stereotypes of them as a "set-in-their-ways" group. Many educational institutions offer courses at reduced or free tuition. Universities and colleges offer short courses during the summer under an international Elderhostel program. Among those attending, many new friendships are formed, and an occasional romance leads to marriage. These courses attract persons who have long been interested in study in a special field, but whose work or family commitments interfered with study earlier.

The disengagement from activities, even from friends and loved ones, considered to be a natural phenomenon of aging, is being challenged by recent research findings which suggest that when this occurs, it may be related more to environmental factors than aging.

The mentally healthy form an increasingly significant segment of society. Their most important contribution may be as teachers and role models to younger persons as they move inevitably toward membership in the elderly population. The Foster Grandparents program sponsored in many communities provides an important and rewarding experience for both the young whom they serve and the elderly who sponsor them.

Many mentally healthy elderly persons live in retirement homes, residence hotels, and group-living arrangements that provide meals, housekeeping, and health services. Some of these facilities provide transportation services such as buses or vans for outings, church attendance, and shopping. Many, although not all, members of this group are less active outside the social and communal life of the facility. Their useful contribution to society may be assisting with physically infirm neighbors in the residence, preparing materials for fund-raising projects, or serving as telephone liaison people for organizations in which they have been active. Their recreation, unlike the travelers who venture to distant places, is likely to be limited to study groups, TV programs, cards and other games, church attendance, reading, and an occasional outing in the community. Ideally, health services for this group are structured to provide consultation, supervision, and emergency intervention. These services are increasingly being supplied by nurse practitioners who conduct in-house clinics and/or visit individual residents on a regular schedule. Many of these residence facilities employ high school and college students or use volunteers from church and community youth groups to serve the evening meal. The contacts are pleasant and stimulating for the elderly, and serve to offer the youth involved insight into the aging process—a lesson of potential value in their own later years.

The elderly with substantial infirmities who continue to live in their own homes are subjected to stresses that range from mere inconveniences to significant hazards to both mental and physical health. They may live alone or with an elderly spouse, mother, family member, or a friend on a marginal income or in a state of poverty. Added to the emotional stress associated with fear of illness, loss of loved ones, and dependency, most of them suffer one or more chronic disabling diseases. They frequently rely on television advertisements and the advice of friends for choices of medicine to relieve health problems. Their ailments may also be complicated by haphazard or excessive use of prescribed drugs and alcohol. They may suffer from drug interactions that result from overuse of prescribed drugs.

The ability of the infirm elderly to cope with seemingly overwhelming problems of daily living is greatly enhanced by a range of community services when these are available. These services include transportation to shop, to conduct essential business, to visit clinics or physicians, to attend church, and to go on occasional outings. Meals-on-wheels and health instruction and supervision by community nursing services and homemaker services are available at modest cost in many communities. If one member of a couple living at home is an invalid, a worker who is available by the hour can relieve the other member to attend to shopping or other errands.

An undetermined number of elderly persons living alone have sensory defects such as hearing loss, limited vision, and memory lapse. Special devices are available to increase the telephone volume. A daily "checkup" on medication and meals by a neighborhood health worker can be done by telephone or by a visit. If an elderly person who lives alone has family or loving friends nearby who visit often, this may be more important than having planned activities.

If the elderly person is on medication, it is useful to initiate a chart system that is kept with the medication to check off the time and date the medicine was taken. Many elderly persons have difficulty with childproof tops on medicine containers. They place medicine in unlabeled containers, creating an additional hazard. Failure to take medicine or taking too much may be a form of suicide intent. The diabetic patient is especially prone to depression, and failures to take insulin or to eat may be deliberate rather than an accident or the result of a memory lapse. The community health worker should be aware of this possibility and evaluate the potential health hazard if there is cause for concern.

Elderly persons may have long-established food preferences that are in conflict with diet needs and restrictions. Dietary education should begin early in life, but it is possible to help elderly persons modify eating habits.

Patience and understanding, as well as assistance with menu planning is sometimes necessary. Assistance with shopping and easy access to appropriate food items (for example, placement on convenient shelves) may be helpful.

The health service worker's goal must be to assist those who need services to maintain a sense of pride and security in their ability to cope, even in a minimal way, as long as this is preferred and possible. However, the health worker should be alert to uncontrolled hazards, be knowledgeable about emergency resources if needed, and be aware of the need for appropriate referral to an authoritative source for further action.

A disturbing development receiving public attention recently is that of abuse of the elderly in their homes. This may be by relatives, neighbors, or others. These abuses may involve physical abuse—even crimes—or harassment to obtain money, the theft of valuables, or damage to property. Any mention of these problems by an elderly person should be reported for investigation by legal and health authorities. Elderly persons who venture out alone to neighborhood shopping centers are all too often victims of purse snatchings.

THE MENTALLY ILL ELDERLY

Organic Mental Disorders (DSM-III) may occur in the presenile period, but are generally associated with persons over 65 years of age. Many of these individuals remain at home with full-time nursing care or care by family members for varying periods of the illness. Others are admitted to nursing homes, geriatric centers, and state psychiatric hospitals when the illness occurs. Organic mental disorders include *dementias* caused by (1) certain *neurologic diseases* and (2) *substance-induced mental disorders.*

The dementias caused by neurologic diseases are generally characterized by confusion, impairment of memory, judgment defects, reduced intellectual functioning, and impairment of orientation.

Alzheimer's disease, first diagnosed by a German physician in 1906, may occur as early as middle age, but may also appear as late as 80. The insidious onset of the dementia follows a progressive course. Changes in personality and behavior as well as loss of memory, intellect, and judgment are apparent, although behavior during the early stages is usually socially acceptable.

In familiar settings, these individuals are usually able to retain contact with family and friends during the early stages. They are frequently frustrated by loss of memory, but they should be encouraged to continue familiar activities. The use of alcohol should be avoided, but no restrictions on diet are indicated.

There is no presently known treatment that effectively interrupts the progressive course of the disease, but medications may be effective in reducing stress and anxiety. In the final stages all ability for self-care is lost. Family members and friends are not recognized.

Huntington's chorea is a hereditary disease affecting members of each generation of a family. The onset generally occurs in the presenile period, usually the late thirties or early forties. During early stages, mood swings from apathy to irritability with occasional delusions are common. As the disease progresses, jerking and flailing movements, grimacing, difficulty in swallowing, and lip smacking are present. These movements can usually be controlled by medication during the early stages, allowing patients to remain at home for varying periods. Someone trained in first aid when choking occurs should always be present during meals. Profound helplessness and dementia mark the final stages. Some of these patients are at suicide risk during the early stages.

Patients who suffer severe *cerebral vascular disease* are often impaired physically and mentally. They are frequently confined to wheelchairs. Sensory losses are evident, and diminished control of bowel and bladder functions may cause distress. These patients require a special quality of nursing care that includes consistent attention to physical deficits. Many patients complain of being cold even on a fairly warm day. The quality of life can also be enhanced by a planned program of socialization and appropriate recreational activities. Family members should be encouraged to visit, even if the patient seems only dimly aware of their identity.

Example: A member of the auxiliary of a geriatric unit in a state hospital and a group of college students were assisting with a Valentine ice cream social for patients. The students had dressed in clown costumes for this event. One unit of the facility housed patients most of whom were in bed or in wheelchairs. As members of the group were serving patients in one area, they met a lively elderly gentleman accompanied by middle-aged children and teenage grandchildren. They were carrying a decorated cake to celebrate, with the frail wife, mother, and grandmother, the sixty-third wedding anniversary of this couple. What a joyous time for the family. The mother appeared to recognize her family, but did not talk. She obviously enjoyed the attention, including the family picture-taking session with the clowns. It was a touching scene, illustrating the principle of preserving and maintaining the quality of life.

A program initiated by a psychiatric nurse employed by a geriatric center is that of using tape-recorded messages from family members and friends, appropriately called "Voices from Loved Ones," to stimulate elderly patients' interest in recalling pleasant memories of past events.

Elderly patients admitted to nursing homes, geriatric centers, and psychiatric hospitals whose conditions are caused by *substance abuses* may present symptoms of acute psychoses, such as hallucinations and delusions. They also have usually neglected nutritional needs. These patients will often respond to a treatment program that includes physical rehabilitation, including nutritional supplementation and medication.

Many of the elderly patients in public psychiatric hospitals were admitted in their youth or middle years with *functional psychoses.* Some have no near relatives or have severed ties with relatives and friends many years ago. These patients are oriented and view the institution as home. Many are infirm, and so have long depended on institutional staff members to shop for personal items, such as shaving cream, snacks, and cosmetics.

Example: The Volunteer and Activities Services directors and Auxiliary members of the center (with administrative support) obtained a shopping cart and equipped it with items frequently requested by patients. The "store," manned by volunteers including high school and college students, makes routine visits to the center. Patients in the center arrive at the "corner store" by wheelchair or walking-cane support, and are aided by the staff to do their weekly shopping. Occasionally a patient purchases a "sample" of a snack, and then goes for a supply when the sample pleases.

Another group of elderly mentally ill are recent admissions to the geriatric centers of mental health systems, nursing homes, or psychiatric hospitals. They must be evaluated for physical ailments, nutritional deficiencies, and other disabling conditions, such as deprivation as a result of extreme isolation. When they are placed on a health-maintaining and health-supporting regimen, some of these patients are able to return to a foster home or a community facility that provides supervision and support from official and voluntary agency personnel. There are increasing numbers of mental health programs and voluntary organizations that sponsor and/or support instructional, social, and recreational activities in which the elderly have opportunities to acquire or improve skills in daily living and make new friends. Such programs may be established as *day-care centers* or as *clubs by community agencies,* assisted by volunteer groups. These centers also serve as an important resource for aged persons who may not be safely left at home when all family members are at work. They need constant or close supervision, but they are able to remain at home with relatives at night and on weekends when family members are at home. This allows family ties to remain intact and serves to keep an elderly person active and more content.

NURSING CONSIDERATIONS

The nursing care requirements of the elderly are similar in many aspects to patients with similar behavior or physical health problems. The elderly in nursing homes, geriatric centers, or community facilities also require some special services and activities to live in dignity and comfort. These include:

- Maintenance of security and dignity and reinforcement of independence to the fullest extent appropriate to the patient's condition.
- Maintenance of the patient's orientation: name of the place, clock, calendar, and daily schedule in a convenient location.
- Encouragement of friendship and communication with staff and other patients.
- Arrangements for patients with visual defects to have assistance for safety.
- Staff members should speak clearly, slowly, and firmly to patients with hearing loss.
- If the patient suffers a painful condition, be especially sensitive to the need for medication to relieve pain.
- Special attention to depression that may reach a stage of suicide risk when a personal or health crisis occurs.
- Observation of any specific interest in an activity reported to a staff member in the activities department.
- Observation of eating habits, especially for food likes and dislikes, difficulty in chewing, or any fixed ideas about food. Report these to the dietitian.
- Report complaints about dentures so that patients can be seen by a dentist. Provide opportunity for women to visit a beauty parlor and see that facial hair is shaved or trimmed.
- Compliment patients on dress and grooming and on any accomplishment. Keep promises to patients faithfully. Under no circumstances assume that "they won't remember anyway."

The elderly in our society who are physically and/or mentally impaired require a comprehensive program of treatment, nursing care, and activities to sustain the quality of life deserved by those whose years of productivity have ceased, but whose interest in life remains. The following is one example of the type of program these citizens deserve.

ACTIVITIES FOR INSTITUTIONALIZED ELDERLY PERSONS*

Many elderly persons who suffer mental and physical impairment spend their later years in institutions. The following summary of the activities department program of the Hancock Geriatric Treatment Center, Williamsburg, Virginia is an example of a comprehensive approach to engaging the skills and interest of patients, and collaboration among health personnel of the center.

The *objectives* of the program are:

To provide a varied assortment of therapeutic, social, and leisure activities designed to meet the needs and interests of the patients.

To build on the skills and interests that patients have retained.

To help patients develop new interests and skills.

Assessment of the status of patients' interests and abilities utilizes a variety of small-group interaction that may include such activities as discussing current events, choir practice, and exercise classes. Nurses, social workers, and other members of the center's staff share information about patients that contributes to planning and the achievement of their objectives.

The *philosophy* is based on the belief that every person needs others and that a person's life is enriched by participation in planning and engaging in activities that help others.

> *Example:* On the day of the interview at the Hancock Geriatric Treatment Center, patients were serving strawberry ice cream and shortcake to infirm patients. The patients had picked the berries on a neighboring farm. In addition to providing a treat for the infirm patients, these patients picked and sold berries to members of the staff.

Patients have their own preferences. They are unwilling to engage in an activity that staff members consider therapeutic, social, or leisure unless it is of interest. One man ignored efforts to interest him in activities until the center acquired a "pet project." He now tends the pets efficiently and with enthusiasm. Patients respond to expectations. A patient who was reminded

---

*Mrs. Alice Richwine, O.T.R., is Director of the Hancock Geriatric Treatment Center Program, Williamsburg, Virginia. This summary is based on an interview with Mrs. Richwine.

that staff members really expected participation in activities did so, reluctantly at first, but later acknowledged that "This sure beats sitting."

The emphasis in the program focuses on small-group interaction, to assist patients who display a need to relearn social skills. Practice may initiate focus on conversation with another. Some patients practice remembering a neighbor's name and respond to an assignment to come to the next group session with the name of a friend.

The following is a list of some of the center's activities:

Remotivation and reminiscence sessions not only help to recall the patient's earlier experiences, but facilitate friendship based on mutual interests and experiences. An example: a small group of men were engaged in a lively discussion about the management of dairy farms, their previous occupations.

Exercise groups help to maintain the patient's mobility and improve circulation.

Therapeutic, social, and leisure activities include:

A trip to a restaurant for lunch (the patient orders from the menu and pays for lunch).

Shopping for purchase of personal items.

Bus rides to observe changes in the area.

Visits to public and/or private recreation centers.

Visit to theme parks.

Involvement in community activities, such as senior citizen organizations in the area.

Day camping.

Participation in the Golden Olympics.

Senior prom in formal dress.

Programs to keep patients involved in news and events in home communities.

Preparation of items for sale in occupational therapy shops.

Regressed patients receive sensory stimulation by touching objects, shaking hands with others, identifying various odors, and listening to music.

Patients serve the center as registered volunteers who participate in a variety of activities to assist other patients. They push patients in wheelchairs to attend events, such as religious services, socials, and games. They fill Easter baskets for the patients, stuff Christmas stockings, and package gifts. They read to and play games with other patients.

LEARNING ACTIVITIES

1. Survey the resources in your community for institutional, community, and home health services to elderly citizens. Present your findings in a class discussion and prepare a list of additional services needed.
2. Interview two elderly persons whom you consider mentally healthy. Identify the concepts that you believe mark them as mentally healthy. You might wish to ask them to share their most rewarding and most threatening experiences with the class and tell how they responded to these experiences.
3. Select an elderly patient for special study and outline a comprehensive program that you believe will enhance this person's achievement of full health potential. Identify health team members who will be involved? What will you expect each representative to contribute to the plan?
4. There are many television programs, brochures, and newspaper and magazine articles that deal with the health, social, and economic problems of the elderly. Report your evaluation of the usefulness, to an elderly person, of a sample program. Ask an elderly person of your acquaintance to share an opinion of a specific publicity account of an activity or program the person has seen.
5. Assume you are responsible for deciding the future care of an elderly confused and infirm grandparent. List the steps you would take and the alternatives you would consider. Explain the reasons for your choice.
6. You have been assigned to membership on a team developing a reality orientation plan for a group of patients. Prepare an outline of the plan that can serve as a basis for charting progress in achieving the treatment objectives. Summarize, at least twice, the progress you observed in a patient's orientation.
7. Look for an elderly person who appears dejected and uninterested in activities and surroundings. Talk with this person and identify what you believe would strike a note of interest and promote involvement in some activity. Use the nursing process as a basis for your plan.

BIBLIOGRAPHY

AMERICAN PSYCHIATRIC ASSOCIATION: *Diagnostic and Statistical Manual of Mental Disorders (DSM-III)*. The Association, Washington, DC, 1980.

BUTLER, RN AND LEWIS, MI: *Aging and Mental Health,* ed 2. CV Mosby, St Louis, 1977.

CARTER, FM: *Psychosocial Nursing,* ed 3. Macmillan, New York, 1981.

HAZARD, M AND KEMP, RE: *Keeping the well elderly well.* Am J Nurs 83: 567–569, April, 1983.

Is America ready for its' elderly? Parade Magazine, Jan 2, 1983, p 12.

THE NATIONAL INSTITUTE ON AGING: *Alzheimer's Disease.* Reprinted by Alzheimer's Disease and Related Disorders Association, Inc. Distributed by The Collaborative Case-Control Study of Alzheimer's Disease, Chicago, 1983.

NODHTURFT, VL AND SWEENEY, M: *Reality orientation therapy for the institutionalized elderly.* Journal of Gerontological Nursing 8:396–401, July, 1982.

Will past voices snap patients into the present? The Eastern Statesman, Williamsburg, Va, Vol 36, No 1, January, 1983.

Audiovisual

KAPLAN, S: *New Programs for Old People: Geropsychiatric Nursing as a Subspecialty.* Educational Cassette Program, from Century Celebration, "Psychiatric Nursing in Historical Perspective," Sponsored by Journal of Psychosocial Nursing and Mental Health Services and Charles B Slack, Inc, Arlington, Va, 1982.

GLOSSARY [1]

Addiction. Psychologic and physiologic dependence on alcohol or some other drug. A person who is addicted will have withdrawal symptoms when the drug is removed.

Adjustment. Ability to cope with life.

Affect. A person's mood—happy or sad.

*Affective reaction.** An illness that shows itself in mood changes.

Aggression. Going after what is wanted without considering others.

Agitation. Severe restlessness caused by emotions.

Ambivalence. Feeling two ways about the same thing at the same time. Example: Love and hate toward the same person.

Amnesia. A complete and sudden loss of memory.

Anxiety. A deep feeling of dread. Worry about what can or might happen.

Apathy. Indifference, lacking interest or feeling, a "just don't care" feeling.

Assertive behavior. Expressing confidence, trying to get what is wanted without hurting others (respecting the other).

Autism. Thinking that is characterized by preoccupation with self, inner thoughts, fantasies, and distorted ideas.

Autonomy. Being independent, doing things for oneself.

Behavior. Any activity that can be observed.

Behavior modification. Behavior is changed by penalizing or rewarding any individual.

Bisexuality. Sexual attraction to both men and women.

Blocking. The person suddenly forgets what he or she is saying in the middle of a sentence or forgets the name of a friend whom he or she is introducing to another.

Circumstantiality. A manner of speech in which it is difficult to understand the central theme because the speaker never gets to the point.

Cohesiveness. A feeling of togetherness in a group.

Commitment procedure. Legal action that allows confinement of a patient to the psychiatric hospital. It may be voluntary or involuntary.

Compulsion. The person keeps doing the same thing over and over again. Examples: Repetitive hand washing and checking locks on doors numerous times.

Confabulation. The person cannot remember certain facts, so makes up what has happened. It is more or less an unconscious process, not deliberate lying.

Conflict. A disagreement from opposing forces.

Confrontation. To face a person with evidence that what he or she is doing is inappropriate, illegal, or unjustified.

Confusion. Disturbed orientation to time, person, and/or place.

Congenital. Present at birth.

Convulsion. A seizure.

Crisis. A person becomes disorganized when an unusual event occurs and usual methods of problem solving are inadequate. Help is needed to cope with the situation.

Decompensation. The person becomes disorganized because of a breakdown of his or her usual defenses.

Defense mechanism. The way in which a person resolves conflicts and stress resulting from situations that are embarrassing, painful, or threatening. They protect the person from anxiety and are unconscious.

Delirium. An acute psychotic state in which the person may feel scared, restless, anxious, and confused. The person may have hallucinations. Delirium is usually caused by a toxic condition as a result of illness or substance abuse.

Delirium tremens (DTs). A psychotic state that occurs when a person who has been drinking a large amount of alcohol over a long period of time suddenly stops drinking.

Delusion. A fixed, false belief that is not altered by logic and reason. Examples: A person who believes she is the Queen of England or he is Napoleon.

Denial. The mind refuses to believe what is true. Example: An alcoholic will not admit to being alcoholic.

Disorientation. The person is unable to remember who he or she is, where he or she is, or the time and/or date.

Drug abuse. Voluntary use of drug that causes serious problems for the person with family, job, money, health, and/or the law. Misuse of prescription or nonprescription medicine and the use of mood-altering substances are also considered to be drug abuse.

Drug dependence. See definition of *addiction*. This term is used more commonly now than addiction.

ECT (Electroconvulsive therapy). A treatment that passes electrical current through the brain. It is most commonly used in depression.

EEG (Electroencephalogram). A diagnostic study that records the electrical activity of the brain. It does not hurt. It is used to study convulsions.

Elopement. Describes the patient who leaves the hospital without permission or awareness of the staff.

Empathy. The ability to feel what another person feels. Putting oneself in the other person's shoes.

Epilepsy. A disorder characterized by periodic, recurring motor activity or sensory seizures. It is caused by abnormal electrical activity in the brain.

Euphoria. An exaggerated feeling of well-being and voluble speech.

Fantasy. Daydream. The person's own private world which is not based on fact or reality.

Feedback. Information given a person about his or her behavior.

Fixation. An obsessive preoccupation with a thought or action.

Flashbacks. Reliving past experience. Usually associated with drug use.

Flight of ideas. Thoughts come to mind very quickly, but there is very little connection between them.

Functional psychosis or illness. A disorder that has a psychologic cause rather than a physical cause.

Guilt. Feeling badly about something one has done or thought.

Hallucination. Seeing, hearing, smelling, feeling, or tasting something that is not there. The sensation comes from within the person rather than the environment.

Hallucinogen. A drug that can cause hallucinations.

Homosexual. A person who is sexually attracted to a person of the same sex.

Hot line. A telephone crisis counseling service.

Hypochrondriasis. Physical complaints that are without an organic basis.

Id. The unconscious impulses and desires of a person.

Ideas of reference. Incorrect interpretation of events as having personal meaning to one's self.

Illusion. The misinterpretation of a real event. Example: A car backfires, and the person believes he heard a gun shot.

Impotence. Inability of the male to achieve an erection and perform sexually.

Impulsive behavior. Behavior in response to anxiety. Done without thinking.

Incest. Having sexual relations with family members.

Insanity. An old term for mental illness. Used in legal procedures.

Insight. Understanding one's own motives and behavior.

Loose association. An unrelated idea reminds a person of another idea. The person listening does not understand. Conversation in which ideas are unrelated, usually found in schizophrenia.

Magical thinking. The idea that thinking something is the same thing as doing it.

Malingering. Pretending to be ill or hurt to avoid any unpleasant situation. May also be used for personal gain. Example: Declaring injury that examination cannot sustain to collect insurance from an accident.

Masochism. Deriving sexual pleasure from being hurt or mistreated by another.

Manipulation. Getting someone to do what you want when the person would not usually plan or offer to do it.

Masturbation. Stroking or touching one's own genitals for pleasure.

Mental status. A standardized procedure for evaluating a patient's psychologic functioning. It includes such factors as appearance, memory, mood, abstractive ability, and intelligence.

Milieu. The environment. In milieu therapy, it is the belief that the environment influences behavior. The aim of a milieu therapy program is to modify the patient's behavior in a positive way.

Mutism. A condition of inability to speak because of an emotional instead of a physical problem.

Neologism. A made-up word, characteristic of patients with schizophrenic disorders.

Neurotic. A person whose problems are caused by a chronic state of anxiety.

Obsession. A persistent, unwanted idea or thought that the individual cannot eliminate by his or her own efforts.

Occupational therapist. A professional who uses purposeful, creative, manual activities to assist the patient. The production of useful articles enhances the person's sense of accomplishment.

Panic. A sudden, overpowering fright caused by anxiety.

Passive-aggressive. A way of expressing anger and hostility by not doing what is wanted or expected. A purposeful inefficiency.

Pedophilia. Achieving sexual satisfaction by using children as sexual objects.

Perception. The way a person views individuals and events.

Personality. All of the thoughts, feelings, and behaviors that makes each person a unique individual.

Perversion. Sexual deviation.

Phobia. A persistent, strong fear of a situation or object that is usually not dangerous.

Psychiatric aide. The title used to identify a person employed to assist with the nursing care of patients. Training may be provided by the employing institution or agency, or in a vocational technical school.

Psychiatric clinical nurse specialist. A graduate of a master's program in the area of psychiatric/mental health nursing. May be certified by the American Nurses' Association.

Psychiatric nurse. A nurse employed in a psychiatric setting. The American Nurses' Association states "a registered nurse in a psychiatric setting who possesses a minimum of a bachelor's degree."

Psychiatric social worker. A graduate of a master's program in social work with special preparation to work with psychiatric patients. The worker deals primarily with the social problems of patients.

Psychiatrist. A physician who has advanced training in psychiatry.

Psychoanalysis. An approach to the treatment of mental illness based on the theories of Sigmund Freud.

Psychoanalyst. A physician who has had psychoanalytic training.

Psychodrama. The use of theater (characters, script, and setting) as a form of therapy. Patients and staff members assume roles cast to concentrate on problems associated with maladaptive behavior.

Psychogenic. Psychologic cause. Not due to an organic disorder.

Psychologist. Specialist in giving and interpreting intelligence and personality tests, who may also do counseling in the prevention and treatment of mental illness. A psychologist does not give medication.

Psychosis. A severe impairment in reality testing. Major problems are disordered thinking and difficulties in communication. A major mental illness.

Recreational therapist. A person who plans, implements, and assists the patient with leisure interests. An objective is that of assisting patients with learning to use their leisure in a healthy manner.

Regression. A defense mechanism in which the person reverts to more childlike forms of behavior.

Remission. A condition in which a patient with a disorder usually considered chronic is without obvious symptoms.

Resistance. Anything that interferes with therapy. May be conscious or unconscious.

Role playing. A therapeutic technique in which one person acts out the part of another person.

Sadism. Getting sexual pleasure from inflicting physical or mental pain on another.

Scapegoating. A term mostly used in family therapy. The blame for all the family difficulties is placed on one member.

Secondary gain. Benefits a person gets from being ill, such as attention, freedom from responsibility, or perhaps money from a disability claim.

Self-concept. The way in which a person thinks about himself or herself. Includes physical and psychologic characteristics.

Self-esteem. The value an individual places upon himself or herself.

Senile dementia. An organic brain disorder of elderly persons causing them to act in a childish manner. Judgment is usually impaired.

Sibling. A brother or a sister.

Significant others. People who are important to the patient.

Stigma. A mask of shame.

Stress. Something that causes tension which creates anxiety.

Suicide. Taking one's own life.

Superego. Commonly called a person's conscious. It usually reflects the values taught by parents and the rules of society.

Therapeutic. Something that causes change and improvement.

Thought disorders. An illness in which a person's thoughts may not be connected and may be delusional, bizarre, or incorrect.

Tranquilizer. A medication given to reduce anxiety.

Voyeur. A person who gets sexual satisfaction by watching others dress or undress or perform sexually.

APPENDICES

APPENDIX 1   EXAMPLE OF PATIENT'S BILL OF RIGHTS*

Except as may be limited on the basis of legal incompetence as adjudicated by a court of competent jurisdiction, each person admitted to a hospital or other facility operated, funded, or licensed by the Department shall:

1. Retain his legal rights as provided by State and Federal law;

2. Receive prompt evaluation and treatment or training about which he is informed insofar as he is capable of understanding;

3. Be treated with dignity as a human being;

4. Not be the subject of experimental or investigational research without his prior written and informed consent or that of his guardian or committee;

5. Be afforded an opportunity to have access to consultation with a private physician at his own expense and, in the case of hazardous treatment or irreversible surgical procedures, have, upon request, an impartial review prior to implementation, except in case of emergency procedures required for the preservation of his health;

6. Be treated under the least restrictive conditions consistent with his condition and not be subjected to unnecessary physical restraint and isolation;

7. Be allowed to send and receive sealed letter mail;

8. Have access to his medical and mental records and be assured of their confidentiality but, notwithstanding other provisions of law, such right shall be limited to access consistent with his condition and sound therapeutic treatment and;

9. Have the right to an impartial review of violations of the rights assured under this section and the right to access to legal counsel.

---

*From Eastern State Hospital, Williamsburg, Virginia, with permission.

APPENDIX 2   *LIST OF COMMUNITY AGENCIES AND ORGANIZATIONS**

Agency on Aging
Al-Anon
Al-Teen
Alcoholics Anonymous
Alzheimer's Disease and Related Disorders Association
Churches
Community Mental Health Center
Contact
Crisis Counseling Agency
Department of Rehabilitative Services
Health Department
Hospital Emergency Departments
Hospital Volunteer Departments and Auxiliaries
Hot Line
Lions Club (Eye Care)
Mental Health Association
National Alliance for the Mentally Ill
Neuropsychiatric Society
Pilot Club
Salvation Army
Schizophrenia Foundation
Social Services Department
VA Hospitals—American Legion

---

*Listing compiled by Mrs. Nancy Munnikysen, C.A.V.S., Director of Volunteer Services, Eastern State Hospital, Williamsburg, Virginia. Community service agencies providing assistance are also listed in local telephone directories at the front of the book or in the Yellow Pages under "Social Service Agencies."

APPENDIX 3

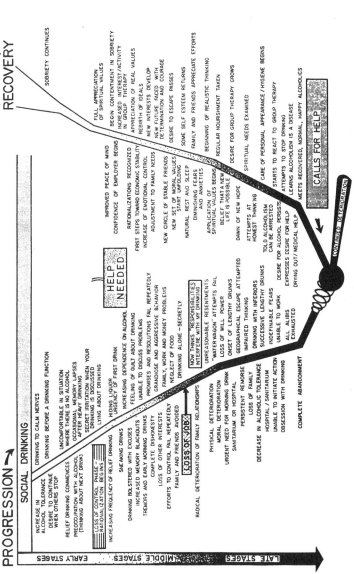

DISEASE of ALCOHOLISM

PROGRESSION →

RECOVERY

SOBRIETY CONTINUES

SOCIAL DRINKING

INCREASE IN ALCOHOL TOLERANCE
DESIRE TO CONTINUE WHEN OTHERS STOP
DRINKING TO CALM NERVES
DRINKING BEFORE A DRINKING FUNCTION

RELIEF DRINKING COMMENCES
UNCOMFORTABLE IN SITUATION WHERE THERE IS NO ALCOHOL
PREOCCUPATION WITH ALCOHOL (THINKING ABOUT NEXT DRINK)
OCCASIONAL MEMORY LAPSES AFTER HEAVY DRINKING
SECRET IRRITATION WHEN YOUR DRINKING IS DISCUSSED
LYING ABOUT DRINKING

LOSS OF CONTROL PHASE — RATIONALIZATION BEGINS

HIDING LIQUOR
URGENCY OF FIRST DRINK
INCREASING FREQUENCY OF RELIEF DRINKING
INCREASING DEPENDENCE ON ALCOHOL
FEELING OF GUILT ABOUT DRINKING
UNABLE TO DISCUSS PROBLEMS
SNEAKING DRINKS
DRINKING BOLSTERED WITH EXCUSES
INCREASED MEMORY BLACKOUTS
PROMISES AND RESOLUTIONS FAIL REPEATEDLY
TREMORS AND EARLY MORNING DRINKS
GRANDIOSE AND AGGRESSIVE BEHAVIOR
COMPLETE DISHONESTY
FAMILY, WORK AND MONEY PROBLEMS
LOSS OF OTHER INTERESTS
NEGLECT OF FOOD
EFFORTS TO CONTROL FAIL REPEATEDLY
DRINKING ALONE — SECRETLY
FAMILY AND FRIENDS AVOIDED

HELP NEEDED

NOW THINKS "RESPONSIBILITIES" INTERFERE WITH MY DRINKING

RADICAL DETERIORATION OF FAMILY RELATIONSHIPS
UNREASONABLE RESENTMENTS
"WATER WAGON" ATTEMPTS FAIL
PHYSICAL DETERIORATION
LOSS OF WILL POWER
MORAL DETERIORATION
ONSET OF LENGTHY DRUNKS
URGENT NEED FOR MORNING DRINK
GEOGRAPHICAL ESCAPE ATTEMPTED
SANITARIUM OR HOSPITAL
IMPAIRED THINKING
PERSISTENT REMORSE
DRINKING WITH INFERIORS
LOSS OF FAMILY
SUCCESSIVE LENGTHY DRUNKS
DECREASE IN ALCOHOLIC TOLERANCE
INDEFINABLE FEARS
HOSPITAL / SANITARIUM
UNABLE TO INITIATE ACTION
UNABLE TO WORK
OBSESSION WITH DRINKING
ALL ALIBIS EXHAUSTED

LOSS OF JOB

COMPLETE ABANDONMENT

IMPROVED PEACE OF MIND
CONFIDENCE OF EMPLOYER BEGINS
BEGIN CONTENTMENT IN SOBRIETY
INCREASED INTEREST / ACTIVITY IN GROUP THERAPY
RATIONALIZATIONS RECOGNIZED
APPRECIATION OF REAL VALUES
FIRST STEPS TOWARD ECONOMIC STABILITY
REBIRTH OF IDEALS
INCREASE OF EMOTIONAL CONTROL
NEW INTERESTS DEVELOP
ADJUSTMENT TO FAMILY NEEDS
NEW FUTURE FACED WITH DETERMINATION AND COURAGE
NEW CIRCLE OF STABLE FRIENDS
DESIRE TO ESCAPE PASSES
NEW SET OF MORAL VALUES START UNFOLDING
SOME SELF ESTEEM RETURNS
NATURAL REST AND SLEEP
FAMILY AND FRIENDS APPRECIATE EFFORTS
DIMINISHING FEARS AND ANXIETIES
BEGINNING OF REALISTIC THINKING
APPLICATION OF SPIRITUAL VALUES BEGINS
REGULAR NOURISHMENT TAKEN
BELIEF THAT A NEW LIFE IS POSSIBLE
DESIRE FOR GROUP THERAPY GROWS
DAWN OF NEW HOPE
SPIRITUAL NEEDS EXAMINED
ATTEMPTS AT HONEST THINKING
CARE OF PERSONAL APPEARANCE / HYGIENE BEGINS
TOLD ALCOHOLISM CAN BE ARRESTED
STARTS TO REACT TO GROUP THERAPY
DESIRE FOR ALCOHOL PERSISTS
ATTEMPTS TO STOP DRINKING
EXPRESSES DESIRE FOR HELP
LEARNS ALCOHOLISM IS A DISEASE
DRYING OUT / MEDICAL HELP
MEETS RECOVERED, NORMAL, HAPPY ALCOHOLICS

FULL APPRECIATION OF SPIRITUAL VALUES

CALLS FOR HELP

CONTINUED DETERIORATION

EARLY STAGES
MIDDLE STAGES
LATE STAGES

(From Glatt, M *Group therapy in alcoholism. Br J Addict* 54:21–28, 1957, with permission.)

INDEX